Reforming the Long-Term-Care System

University Health Policy Consortium Series

In 1977, Boston University, Brandeis University, and the Massachusetts Institute of Technology established the University Health Policy Consortium to conduct health policy analyses and research projects and to provide an educational laboratory for students interested in health policy. A year later, the Health Care Financing Administration designated the Consortium as its first Center for Health Policy Analysis and Research. The Center concentrates its research in three major health-care areas: long-term care, health-care quality and effectiveness, and regulation and reimbursement.

Brandeis University is the host institution for the Consortium, which is housed at the Florence Heller Graduate School for Advanced Studies in Social Welfare. Both the Center and the Consortium bring together social scientists, lawyers, and medical personnel to conduct collaborative research in health care.

This book represents some of the analyses that have been done by the Consortium's associates. It is the first book in the health series to be published by Lexington Books.

Other books in the UHPC series are:

Federal Health Programs
Edited by Stuart H. Altman and Harvey M. Sapolsky

Rural Medicine
Stanley S. Wallack and Sandra E. Kretz

Variations in Hospital Use
Edited by David Rothberg

Reforming the Long-Term-Care System

Financial and Organizational Options

Edited by
James J. Callahan, Jr.
Stanley S. Wallack
University Health Policy
Consortium

Research supported by the
Health Care Financing Administration
Office of Research, Demonstrations,
and Statistics

LexingtonBooks
D.C. Heath and Company
Lexington, Massachusetts
Toronto

Library of Congress Cataloging in Publication Data

Main entry under title:
 Reforming the long-term-care system.

 1. Long-term care of the sick—United States—Administration. 2. Long-term care of the sick—United States—Finance. 3. Medical policy—United States.
I. Callahan, James J. II. Wallack, Stanley.
RA644.6.R45   362.1'6'068   80-8366
ISBN 0-669-04040-1

Published simultaneously in Canada

Printed in the United States of America

International Standard Book Number: 0-669-04040-1

Library of Congress Catalog Card Number: 80-8366

Contents

Foreword

The mission of the Health Care Financing Administration (HCFA) of the Department of Health and Human Services is to promote the timely delivery of appropriate, quality health care to its beneficiaries—approximately 45 million aged, disabled, and poor Americans. These people constitute the most vulnerable members of our society.

As part of that mission, HCFA will spend $15 billion of its $42 billion budget on long-term care in fiscal 1980. Total public funds spent for long-term care during the same period will be $21.6 billion. These costs are projected to grow to $42 billion by 1985 and to $75.6 billion by 1990, only ten years in the future. Recent expenditures on long-term care have grown and are expected to grow at a more rapid rate than any other expenditure in the health-care sector.

As the authors of this volume point out, the root of the long-term-care problem lies in a social situation that the United States has not heretofore experienced. In recent years, increased life expectancy and declining birth rates have led to a greater number of people living into old age than ever before. Furthermore, our population has become much less able to care for dependent adults because of increased mobility, weakening of the nuclear family, and entry of many women (our major caregivers in the past) into the paid-labor market.

Such rapid social change has required increased public awareness, expectations, and expenditures. Yet experience has shown that, in many areas of the public sector, the forces of social change are only imperfectly understood and inadequately addressed. In the learning process, mistakes are inevitably made and are only rectified as we move toward the development of desirable policies.

This volume is a product of HCFA's effort to fund research into what has occurred in the long-term-care area and how we might achieve future improvement in our programs. During the next decade we will be developing a long-term-care system with the goals of helping people to remain as independent as possible and assuring that long-term-care services, both within and outside of institutions, are humane and of high quality. This volume provides worthy insights for our emerging understanding of the key issues and policy options available to us.

Howard N. Newman
Administrator,
Health Care
Financing Administration

Acknowledgments

The compilation of chapters on reforming the long-term-care delivery system was made possible by the cooperative efforts of the authors and other research associates at the University Health Policy Consortium. The authors had to work together, both in the formulation of their own chapters and in the review of each others' work, in order to provide a systematic comparison of the options developed. Financial and intellectual support for these chapters came from the Health Care Financing Administration (HCFA). Judith Williams and Diane Rowland were of particular assistance. This comparison of options was one of the major tasks undertaken in 1979 at the Center for Health Policy Analysis and Research, which was established to conduct policy analysis and research studies relevant to HCFA. The Center's efforts were complemented by funds from the HCFA-funded National Long-Term Care Demonstration Project, which allowed us to include chapters on the Disability Allowance and the Social/Health Maintenance Organization.

The editors would like to thank the authors for their willingness to write their chapters according to specific guidelines and criteria. In the review of these chapters, a number of individuals made valuable contributions. The efforts of Janet Mitchell, Susan Sanders Lehrer, John Drew, R. Hopkins Holmberg, Ralph Berry, Thomas McGuire, and Thomas Willemain greatly improved the content of the various chapters. Robert Morris was instrumental in getting this comparative analysis formulated.

The patience of Natalie Andrews, Mary Smith, Barbara Isaacson, and Marion Rabinowitz in typing the various drafts and of Katherine Raskin in editing the manuscript is appreciated.

Part I
Introduction

1 Major Reforms in Long-Term Care

James J. Callahan, Jr., and
Stanley S. Wallack

Social reforms in the United States are usually characterized as incremental in nature. Ideas for change are proposed, contested, debated, modified, and then grafted on to some existing law or program. Even changes as dramatic as Medicare and Medicaid were built upon the pre-existing programs of Medical Aid to the Aged and vendor payments for welfare recipients. Incremental changes, however, extend along a continuum from major to "tinkering with the system." Major reforms would alter some of the essential features of the system, while tinkering essentially is cosmetic.

The success of a reform, be it major or tinkering, must be measured against the situation or problem it attempts to resolve. At times, no amount of tinkering can approach what observers would agree to be a satisfactory resolution of a problem. Reforms approaching the major point on the continuum are required. Such is the need for reform in the area of long-term care.

Long-term care refers to the financing, organization, and delivery of a wide range of medical and human services to a class of people who are severely disabled or limited in their functional capacities for a relatively long and indefinite period of time. While the United States has been relatively successful in providing medical services to the general population, it has been much less successful in providing the necessary array of services to the mentally and physically chronically ill. The success achieved in the acute care section is due in large part to heavy federal intervention. This intervention has ranged from grant-in-aid programs of the Public Health Service to the massive medical care programs of Medicare and Medicaid. Despite the growth of these medical programs, as well as social service programs (for example, Title XX), over the past twenty years, long-term-care problems remain. Federal involvement has yet to find the appropriate point of intervention in the very complex structure of service to the chronically ill and disabled. State and local governments lack the willingness and capacity to assume the total financial and service responsibility for the population. Long-term care is a very big problem affecting millions of individuals and families and involving the expenditures of billions of dollars.

Estimates indicate that 1.4 million persons with chronic conditions are residing in nursing homes. Estimates of the number of severely disabled

3

in the community range from 3 to 6 million persons. Beyond these individuals are the family members who provide assistance to their disabled kin and, consequently, have to adjust their financing and time budgets to the situation.

Well over $20 billion are spent on this problem by public authorities. Personal out-of-pocket expenditures for long-term care are difficult to estimate but probably approach $10 billion. The cost of family care has been estimated at $38.2 billion by the Comptroller General.

Large numbers of institutions, agencies, and providers are involved in long-term care. Approximately 20,000 nursing homes, 2,300 home health agencies, 40,000 home health aides, plus numerous other providers are involved in care of the disabled.

Despite the many public dollars being spent and the number of organizations available, a litany of long-term-care problems has been identified. Included are the following:

Unmet needs of the disabled continue to persist,

Current programs are biased towards institutionalization,

Quality of care is low,

Benefits are maldistributed geographically,

Public expenditures are rising rapidly,

Services and financing are categorical and fragmented,

Case management is lacking.

These problems, discussed in detail by Morris and Youket in chapter 2, point to the need for timely major reforms in the financing, organization, and delivery of long-term-care services. More tinkering, adding a benefit here, removing a barrier there, will not suffice. The one social invention that was able to provide the broad array of services under one roof—the institution—has lost favor both for economic and humanistic reasons.

No consensus has emerged on how these complex needs should be financed and organized in the community. Fundamental value decisions as to the responsibility of the individual family and various incremental entities need to be sorted out. Pressures are mounting on the government to take some action. The increased responsibility suggested has been expansion into financing, organizing, regulating, and delivering the services. Within these categories, options are available to the government. In the financing area, for example, either cash benefits or categorical program support could be selected. The choice of financing mechanism depends on how much responsibility the individual has vis-à-vis the providers and governmental regulation in determining how much of what resources are purchased. This volume on the financing and organization of care for the physically disabled or functionally limited was designed with this lack of consensus in mind.

Values as well as current problems dictate which set of options should be considered. Part I briefly describes the current state of long-term-care needs, reviews the previous attempts to develop reform proposals, and ends by describing the limitations of these attempts as well as our effort.

The options are presented in Parts II and III. Part II includes financing reforms: bloc grants, compulsory social insurance, and disability allowance. In Part III, the organizational reforms of case management, a single agency, and a Social/Health Maintenance Organization (S/HMO) are prescribed. The last option really goes beyond an organization change, incorporating fixed budgets and a more comprehensive provider than now exists. Part III also describes a systems approach to long-term care and suggests areas worthy of future research.

While six discrete financing and organizational reforms have been constructed, they can be structured so as to be almost indistinguishable from some of the others. For example, a voucher and insurance system are both benefit-delimited programs. A voucher system differs fundamentally from a social insurance program because of the contributory nature of insurance programs. Nevertheless, by the use or nonuse of copayments, delineation of benefits, and eligible providers, the programs could turn out to look quite different. Alternatively, a case management system with strong authority over flow of patients or over resource use, is hard to distinguish from a single agency option.

Efforts have been taken to describe the reforms in general terms, showing how the programs can be altered. Because the form of the option is critical in terms of alleviating certain problems, the major characteristics of each option are described before attempts are made to analyze their impact. While these options have been discussed previously at HCFA and other governmental agencies, they have not been subjected to vigorous comparative analysis. This set of analyses tries to do just that. Before describing the criteria used in this comparative analysis, the global considerations of goals and objectives need to be highlighted.

Goals of Long-Term-Care Services

Any discussion of options must take into account the question: Options for what? An option cannot be evaluated except by matching it against the goal(s) it is presumed to achieve. In the area of long-term care, however, goals have not been well articulated and, when they have been, they are frequently contradictory.

The first level of goals relates to the outcomes to be produced by the long-term-care system (see figure 9-1). The outcome desired for particular individuals will differ according to the individual's characteristics and needs. Five desired goals have been identified:

1. Maximum possible functional independence of an individual at all times, even if there are limitations in activity or deterioration of function;
2. Rehabilitation of an individual, restoring him/her to some previous level of functioning that can be sustained;
3. Humane care for persons who are functionally and permanently dependent;
4. Utilization of the least restrictive environment;
5. Death with dignity for individuals in the dying process.

These outcome goals usually are not mentioned in the long-term-care literature, but they serve as the basic justification for the existence of long-term-care services.

Goals are usually stated at a second level of analysis as well. For example, they may be stated:

To meet all the medical/social needs of the entire long-term-care population;

To provide a coordinated, comprehensive system of care;

To provide equal access to long-term-care services;

To reduce the cost of long-term-care services by more appropriate use of existing resources.

This list could go on and the relative importance of these goals is easily altered. An advocate, for example, may rank meeting all needs as very important, while a budget analyst might rank reducing cost as the first priority. Under these circumstances, each option can be ranked differently.

The contributors to this volume developed the following goals and criteria by which they would evaluate their options to the extent that available information and data permitted.

Specific Criteria Used in Evaluating the Options

1. Coverage
   a. Does option add coverage of people? of services?

    b. Is option based on additional dollars or zero-base reallocation?
2. Effect on consumers
    a. Is access altered for subpopulations?
    b. Is horizontal equity increased—that is, base option gives persons with like needs access to and choice of all services?
    c. Does option alter protection against abuse or neglect?
3. Distribution of costs and their effect
    a. Upon individuals, families, and relatives;
    b. Upon levels of government;
    c. Upon administrative costs: Are they increased or not?
4. Organizational issues
    a. What is the locus of control—user, provider, government, bureaucracy, third parties—as to:
        1. Services used or arranged
        2. Control over demand
        3. Targeting
5. Effect on providers
    a. Shift production of service supply (add new volume with or without more providers);
    b. Alter service supply mix;
    c. Encourage flexible use of services—that is, substitution of one type of service for another;
    d. Shift service supply among different types of providers;
    e. Shift shares of long-term-care-resource allocation.
6. Political and economic feasibility—How will each option handle political issues of
    a. Inflation,
    b. Budget caps,
    c. Constituency pressures.

As previously stressed, the expected results from these major reforms are limited to the explicit form that the reforms finally take. Each option can, theoretically, be shaped to bias the results in favor of institutional care or in-home care through the built-in entitlement or eligibility criteria. For example, the effect on the distribution of costs can be altered by a shift in co-insurance or in federal/state sharing. The distribution of benefits is affected by eligibility according to income, disability level, and family status. Thus, the actual outcome of any one option depends upon the policy choices made with regard to access, benefit distribution, cost sharing, cost containment, and quality-assurance. Nevertheless, fundamental differences exist in the role of consumers, providers, and government; and a financing solution, if made with no organizational reforms, will have very different results than an organizational change taken alone.

Making Decisions and Choices

The financing options—social insurance and disability vouchers—would alter the distribution of expenditures; the management options—a single agency and case management—would better match needs to services; and the S/HMO would combine changes in delivery with those in financing and administration. While the impact of the reform options on existing deficiencies differ, they have one thing in common: they would improve the long-term-care system.

A comparative analysis clarifies how any one option could correct the "system defects" as measured against the probable results of the other options. Since no one reform addresses all of the problems, it is essential that the identified goals be prioritized in order to select the most desirable long-term-care reform(s). In addition, these goals must be matched by an assessment of what is a feasible approach, given existing political and economic realities. For example, the compulsory social insurance system might be judged most powerful, but the pressure on the existing payroll tax structure may render it infeasible. A S/HMO may be the best way to combine financing and delivery in a mechanism that permits the most efficient use of resources. Until this model is tested in different sites as to its ability to enroll elders and provide the full spectrum of care, however, a major national effort appears to be out of the question. Less powerful approaches, such as case management or a single-channeling agency, are now being tested by Washington, but it is questionable as to the ability of these mechanisms to seriously change existing patterns of service. Other approaches such as involving the states in planning to meet the long-term-care needs of their citizens may be more feasible, although suffering the limitations that currently characterize the federal/state relationships.

Different groups or government entities appear to have different goals. Clearly, change in the long-term-care system is warranted, but it will occur only when it is decided who has the responsibility first for leading a change in the system and, secondly, for carrying out the changes. It is unlikely that one level of government will come forward and seek responsibility for all aspects (planning, organizing, delivery, and financing) of the long-term-care system. Rationalizing the role of the different levels of government appears important. The federal government, because of its income and health programs, will undoubtedly continue to be the major financier; the states, because of their social-services programs, will continue to have the responsibility for coordinating the federal and state efforts; and the delivery of services will continue to involve local governments and private providers.

A Need for Federal Leadership

Action at the federal level is paramount since major changes in the long-term-care system and in the current patterns of care necessitate some changes in the way the long-term-care system is financed. In order to improve the matching of services and needs, payment for the necessary services must occur. The most appropriate method for changing the financing of long-term care is, however, unknown. Given this fact and the potential for large expenditure increases, "experiments" should occur with different financial reforms. To accomplish financial reforms requires federal action. The Federal Department of Health and Human Services is now considering what "experimental" systems will be tried in the 1980s.

The financial and organizational reforms selected at the federal and state levels will largely establish whether the delivery system will be private or public. To the extent that individuals are given more control over the total financing of care—whether in the form of cash or benefits—the greater likelihood is that the delivery system at the local level will be private. But if the decision is to make case management the cornerstone of reform without any alteration in financing, then the greater likelihood is that a governmental-type delivery system will evolve.

Since the current federal demonstration effort (known as *channeling*) may be the one opportunity for the federal government to radically alter the long-term-care system, a broad array of financing experiments should be considered. The experiments should consider organizational reforms, cash and benefit approaches, bloc grants and S/HMOs. The unlikelihood of having additional federal dollars made available for new long-term-care programs in the 1980s must make one cognizant of the financial resources—at various governmental levels—that will be potentially available to the elderly. As the age structure of this nation shifts over the next thirty or forty years and the proportion of the elderly relative to the working population rises, ways must be found to use the public dollars allocated to the aged more efficiently.

What is required to move ahead is the combination of goals selection and priorities, decisions as to the level of government responsible for different aspects of the long-term-care system, testing of new ideas, and a thorough discourse on the problems and needs of persons requiring personal care from others over a prolonged period of time. Discourse without benefit of knowledge on the consequences of policy changes may bring frustration. Analysis conducted by experts, without benefit of the hopes and goals of those to be affected, may bring empty results. The fact is that, at this very moment, literally millions of people are coping in one way or another with problems of long-term care. Public officials at all levels of government, for good or ill, are making decisions affecting the lives of people. Providers are delivering services, some of unknown quality and with mixed results. The authors hope that this volume will contribute to a constructive dialogue on future directions in long-term care in this country.

2 The Long-Term-Care Issues: Identifying the Problems and Potential Solutions

Robert Morris and
Paul Youket

The problems of the long-term-care system have changed since the first major treatment of the subject was undertaken by the Commission on Chronic Illness (1956). If anything, they have been more intensive, making the necessary reforms more expensive and difficult to accomplish. First, the policy of incremental changes pursued over the past twenty years increased the number of programs, with special interest groups organized by age, condition, disability level, and so forth. Developing coalitions without doing harm to some groups has, therefore, become more difficult. A medical system that serves the acute care health problems has flourished, independently of the locally-based social service system. Neither system claims responsibility for the long-term-care patient whose needs span both systems. Buck passing persists in this environment, which has not developed appropriate linkages.

Secondly, increase in longevity and the growth of the population in toto means that more individuals have chronic physical illnesses that hinder their capacity to function. Today, these are estimated to be between 3 and 6 million persons outside of institutions, and over 3 million family units provide major physical, personal, or financial help to their disabled elderly living outside of institutions. In addition, 20,185 nursing care institutions with 1,407,000 beds and over 2,350 home care agencies are directly involved in providing care, along with an estimated 25 percent of acute hospital care devoted to the acute episodes of illness encountered by the long-term population.

Despite large and growing expenditures (over $20 billion in 1978), publicly funded programs appear peripheral against the background of the informal helping system made up of relatives and friends. An estimated 70 percent of elderly rely mainly on relatives to meet their personal- and physical-care needs in case of disability rather than on agencies. In some studies, the elderly use the informal support system in five cases for each case using an organized agency service. The persons depending on the formal support systems are more likely to be without relatives, to be much older, and to be much poorer—although the overlap between the two

11

groups is substantial. In cases involving children and young adults, the proportion relying upon the informal system is even higher (Gurland 1978; Branch 1978; Eggert et al. 1977; Klerman 1978).

Past Efforts to Define a Federal Policy

Long-term-care needs have grown and the system has taken on increased complexity because of the indifference at the federal level. National debate about health insurance, which culminated in enactment of Titles XVIII and XIX of the Social Security Act, focused attention between 1957 and 1965 on acute illness. Caring in a similar manner for the chronically ill was not seen as a federal responsibility. Not until the 1970s did long-term care again become a major object of public policy attention, for at least two reasons: (1) escalating public expenditures for health care perturbed the Social Security system, the basic health-care system, and public officials; and (2) a confusing proliferation of specialized programs was established to deal with parts of the long-term-care problem, but which introduced confusion into both health and welfare systems. Thus, the federal government has backed into a position of being concerned with chronic illness, if only to orchestrate the necessary changes.

In the early 1970s, an accumulation of studies explained why some major reform is needed, and a number of policy analyses attempted to sift out the most promising approaches (see appendix). These studies and analyses have been insufficient for the adoption of a new approach, but their findings need to be reviewed, for they provide the foundation on which the present analysis is based.

Summary of Arguments Advanced for Changes in Current Arrangements—The Problem of Long-Term Care

Arguments advanced for changing current arrangements can be summed up as follows:

Persistence of unmet needs in the population,

Bias toward institutionalization,

Low levels of the quality of care produced,

Geographical inequity and maldistribution of benefits,

Excessive burdens placed on families,

Rapidly rising public and private expenditures,

Fragmentation among services and financing,

Lack of case management functions.

An understanding of these arguments is useful in analyzing what the various options for change can be expected to produce. Each of these arguments is discussed in the following sections.

Unmet Needs

It is commonly said that the present system of long-term care fails to meet many of the needs of those who require some form of long-term care, particularly those with needs for noninstitutional services. The U.S. Department of Health, Education and Welfare (HEW) (1978, p. 3 and appendix 10, table 1) states that 3.6 to 7.8 million disabled adults receive no formal long-term-care services; some of these persons, however, are receiving informal care through family or friends. The Congressional Budget Office (CBO) estimates that in 1976 up to 1.4 million disabled adults who were living alone received no care, either formal or informal; no estimates were made, however, on what proportion of these persons did not, in fact, require any care by others (CBO 1977a, pp. 16-17). The CBO does estimate that "3 to 5 percent of the total noninstitutionalized population (12 to 17 percent of the elderly) have levels of disability so high that they are bedridden or require assistance in the most basic functions of daily living. . . ."; many of these persons may, in fact, require some level of institutional care (CBO 1977a, p. 20).

The CBO also estimates that in 1976 the number of adults needing to live in personal care homes, sheltered living arrangements, and congregate housing exceeded the number actually residing in such facilities by more than 1.1 million. By 1985, they estimate that 1.1 to 1.3 million adults will have unmet needs for personal care homes, sheltered living arrangements, and congregate housing. Similarly, they estimate that in 1976 1.4 to 2.2 million more adults needed home health care or day care than the number served. By 1985, they estimate that 2.9 to 4.3 million adults will have unmet needs for home-based services (CBO 1977a, pp. 20 and 45).

Such evidence about need is flawed in several ways: (1) the criteria are often ambiguous; (2) the basis for government provision does not distinguish well between governmental, family, and local community care now provided; (3) the data do not permit clear targeting of priority cases if funds are to be very limited; if funds were to be much increased, the data do not permit very accurate predictions about how patients would in fact use whatever services are offered or about how they would respond to expert judgments about what services they should use; (4) degrees of severity or of suffering are not identified, so that patient wants are not distinguished from assessed needs nor are real behavioral choices of patients and families distinguished from opinions expressed in surveys. The CBO estimates are useful as rough preliminary guides, not as firmly rooted ones.

If one of the objectives of long-term-care reform is to eliminate all of these unmet needs, then eligibility and benefits under public programs providing resources for long-term care, as well as the actual supply of noninstitutional long-term-care services, would have to be greatly expanded. This could be done under existing programs, but doing so would raise public costs for long-term care substantially and would substitute formal care for informal care and public payment for services for private payment for services.

Bias toward Institutional Care

It is also said that the present system of long-term care is strongly biased in favor of institutional care and places little emphasis on care in community settings. The CBO estimates that over 90 percent of all public expenditures for long-term care go for institutional care (CBO 1977a, p. 14). Medicaid is the primary source of public funding for long-term care. In fiscal year (FY) 1978, 38 percent of total Medicaid expenditures was spent on institutional long-term-care services, while only 0.8 percent of total Medicaid expenditures was spent on home health services (HEW 1978, appendix 10, table 2).

With most public money for long-term care flowing into institutional care, many persons with some needs for long-term care are unnecessarily or inappropriately institutionalized so that they can receive the needed public support for their care. Estimates from empirical studies of the proportion of nursing home residents inappropriately placed range from 6 percent to 76 percent (CBO 1977a, pp. 55-56). The CBO concludes, on the basis of these studies, that at least 10 to 20 percent of all skilled nursing facility (SNF) patients and 20 to 40 percent of all intermediate care facility (ICF) residents are probably receiving unnecessarily high levels of care (CBO 1977a, p. 18). HEW (1978, p. 3) estimates "that between 14 and 25 percent of institutionalized patients could be cared for in less restrictive settings (though not necessarily less expensively)."

Insufficient supplies of community care services and restrictions under present public programs are the reasons most frequently cited for the overutilization of institutional care services and the underutilization of community care services. Personal care services are necessary in many cases to maintain individuals with long-term-care needs in community settings. Services covered under Medicaid must be "medically related." States can reimburse personal care and day care services under Medicaid but few do so. Most funding for such services is through Title XX. While Medicaid is an open-ended, federal/state matching program, Title XX is a close-ended, federal/state matching program. In FY 1980, Medicaid is estimated to spend $8.4 billion on long-term-care services, 98 percent of which will be used for institutional long-term-care services, while in the same year Title XX is estimated to spend only $574 million on noninstitutional services for the elderly and disabled (HEW 1978, appendix 10, table 4).

Another factor that works to bias public coverage of long-term care in favor of institutional care is the way in which persons become eligible for Medicaid. In states that cover the "medically needy," expenses for institutional care are often high enough to make many of those who are institutionalized quickly eligible for Medicaid, while expenses for home health services are generally not high enough to make many persons with similar needs eligible for Medicaid. In addition, many restrictions are in force on coverage of home health services under Medicare and Medicaid, which have greatly limited the utilization of these services under these programs (HEW 1978, appendix 2; CBO 1977a, pp. 27-30). Further, social, homemaker, and personal care supports may be excluded from home health programs, although these less medical-type services are seen by consumers as crucial to maintaining life outside a nursing home.

A desire to more equally balance the provision of institutional care and noninstitutional care would require examining the supply and program coverage of noninstitutional-care services. This could be done under present programs, but this approach would probably raise total public costs for long-term care. Public officials are fearful that the increased demand for noninstitutional-care services would outweigh the decreased demand for institutional-care services. The CBO estimates that a federal social-insurance program fully covering all identified institutional and noninstitutional long-term-care service needs would expand both the population entitled to public care and the scope of reimbursed services sufficiently to increase outlays under federal programs by $32.1 to $55.8 billion over present law by 1985 (CBO 1977b, p. 27). The argument to rectify an institutional bias thus encounters a challenge about how to do so *without* expanding entitlements, both to a wider eligible population and a broader range of services.

Poor Quality of Care

A third major source of concern is the quality of care received by many persons within the present system of long-term care. Public scandals of poor quality nursing home care have abounded; widespread instances of poor quality nursing home care have been well documented by such sources as the Subcommittee on Long-Term Care of the U.S. Senate Special Committee on Aging, the New York State Moreland Act Commission, and Mary A. Mendelson in her book, *Tender Loving Greed*. In 1973, the Office of Nursing Home Affairs in HEW found that 59 percent of all nursing home beds did not meet minimum federal standards of quality (HEW 1977, p. 18). According to the 1977 National Nursing Home Survey, 25 percent of all nursing home facilities and 11.9 percent of all nursing home beds are not certified under either Medicare or Medicaid; 10.6 percent of all nursing home residents are in such beds (HEW 1979, p. 8).

HEW (1978, p. 4) cites the heavy use of medications, the administration of drugs by untrained orderlies, the rarity of physician visits, and high staff turnover as indicators of poor quality of care in nursing homes. It also states that anecdotal evidence exists of appalling instances of low quality care "in the provision of unregulated in-home services under Title XX." It attributes this low quality to the lack of federal standards for providers of home-based services under Title XX (HEW 1978, p. 3). It is not known, however, how widespread these problems are for community- and home-based-care services. Measuring the quality of care provided is even more difficult in noninstitutional settings than it is in institutional settings.

HEW (1978) argues that many deficiencies of quality assurance exist for institutional long-term care in the current system. The current system, it says, is "complex, cumbersome, uncoordinated, and often ineffective. Existing mechanisms tend to focus on the physical capacity of the facilities and the appropriateness of the level of care rendered, not on the quality of care received." Present "review mechanisms do not successfully assure that LTC [long-term-care] patients receive adequate and appropriate services to meet their needs. Although we can assess LTC [long-term-care] patients' conditions to determine their degree of debilitation, there is no agreement on what constitutes 'quality of care' in response to their needs." ". . . [O]utcome measures against which quality of care can be assessed must include both medical, functional, and social dimensions, but such measures have not been fully developed" (HEW 1978, p. 1).

HEW (1978) goes on to list many specific problems of the current system for quality assurance of institutional long-term care. It recommends the development of "a single integrated long-term-care quality-assurance system" and specifies many regulatory and legislative changes that should be made in the present system (HEW 1978, appendix 3, p. 3).

Inequality across States and among Consumers

Another problem of concern in the current system of long-term care is the inequity in care resulting from the wide variations in long-term-care services across the states. For example, in 1974-75, the supply of nursing home beds per 1,000 elderly varied from a high of 116.8 in Minnesota to a low of 15.9 in Virginia (HEW 1978, appendix 10, table 7). Expenditures for long-term-care services as a percentage of total state Medicaid expenditures in FY 1977 varied from 13.9 percent in the District of Columbia and 27.1 percent in California to 65.9 percent in South Dakota and 76.7 percent in Alaska. The state of New York alone accounts for 23 percent of all Medicaid expenditures for long-term-care services; the top ten states account for 65 percent of all Medicaid expenditures for long-term care. Similar variations in state expenditures for long-term-care services exist under Title XX as well (HEW 1978, appendix 10, table 17).

These inequalities in long-term care across states are due primarily to the discretion allowed to states in determining eligiblity, benefits, and reimbursement rates under Medicaid and Title XX. In general, larger and more urban states with high per capita incomes spend more for long-term-care services than do smaller and more rural states with low per capita incomes (Correia 1976, p. 27). One cannot assume from this, however, that long-term-care needs are less well met in low-expenditure states and better met in high-expenditure states.

Less quantitative reasons also exist for unease about equity. There is a belief that the present system of public provision has worked out inequitably in the way in which persons with like conditions are treated. For example, some families bear heavy burdens of personal care for their members, and other families succeed easily in shifting care to others; some with minimal loss of mobility are institutionalized, while others with great loss of capacity remain in the community. It is unclear what causes lie behind these perceived inequities.

Heavy Burden on Individuals and Families

The heavy financial burden that individuals and families must bear under the current system of long-term care is another leading reason often cited for the need to change the present system. The costs of long-term care can be financially catastrophic for individuals and families. "According to a CBO analysis of the incidence and cost of illness, nursing home care is the principal cause of catastrophic expenses among the aged." The CBO estimates that "the average annual cost of a nursing home stay in 1975 was $7,300." However, 68 percent of the disabled, 73 percent of the disabled elderly, and 76 percent of the institutionalized population have household incomes below $7,000 a year (CBO 1977a, p. 23).

In FY 1977, 41.4 percent of all national expenditures for nursing home care was paid directly by consumers (Gibson and Fisher 1978). In FY 1976, the CBO estimated that 38 to 44 percent of total national spending for all long-term-care services was paid directly by consumers (CBO 1977b, p. 12).

Medicaid pays for 51 percent of all nursing home care and 28 to 31 percent of all long-term-care services in this country (Gibson and Fisher 1978). In order for individuals to become eligible for Medicaid, however, they must first impoverish themselves. In some states, individuals whose incomes are above the eligibility level can "spend-down" (in terms of their medical expenses) to become eligible for Medicaid (the medically needy). According to the CBO, "47.5 percent of nursing home patients depleted their resources and qualified as 'medically needy'" (CBO 1977a, p. 24). In addition, all Medicaid recipients who are institutionalized must give up all of their income above a personal allowance (generally $25) in order to help pay for the costs of their care.

In order to reduce the financial burden of long-term care on individuals and families, the public share of the costs for long-term-care services would have to be increased.

In addition to financial distress, families and individuals suffer great distress in trying to deal with severe disability without external help. A New York City study found that severe mental depression was found in 25 percent of families with disabled elders (Gurland 1978).

*Uncontrolled Increases in Public
and Private Expenditures*

Major reforms in the present system of long-term care are also needed because of the skyrocketing costs of long-term care. From FY 1965 to FY 1977, national expenditures for nursing home care alone grew from $1.3 billion to $12.6 billion, an increase of 869 percent. In relative terms, national expenditures for nursing home care have grown from 3.3 percent of all national health expenditures in FY 1965 to 7.8 percent of all national health expenditures in FY 1977 (Gibson and Fisher 1978). The CBO estimates total national spending for all long-term-care services to have been $18.1 to $20.4 billion in FY 1976; this would constitute 12.8 to 14.5 percent of total national health expenditures in that year (CBO 1977b, p. 12). These figures do not clarify whether the increases are unreasonable, or represent a shift in medical-cost accounting from acute- to long-term-care cost centers, or represent a delayed response to demographic trends.

This increase in spending for long-term care is partly due to coverage of long-term care services by public programs, particularly by Medicaid. Public programs paid 57 percent of all national expenditures for nursing home care in FY 1977 and 51 to 57 percent of national expenditures for all long-term care services in FY 1976. Medicaid alone paid 51 percent for all national expenditures for nursing home care in FY 1977 and 28 to 31 percent of national expenditures for all long-term-care services in FY 1976 (Gibson and Fisher 1978). HEW (1978) estimates total public spending for long-term care to have been about $12 billion in FY 1977 (HEW 1978, p. 3). Medicaid expenditures for long-term-care services have grown 122 percent from $3.4 billion in FY 1973 to $7.5 billion in FY 1978 (HEW 1978, appendix 10, table 2). HEW (1978, p. 5) contends that Medicaid, as an open-ended, federal/state matching program in which states control eligibility, benefits, and reimbursement under minimum federal requirements, has been chiefly responsible for uncontrolled growth in federal spending for long-term care.

Federal costs for long-term care are expected to continue to grow much higher as a result of the aging of the population and the impact of judicial decisions. The number of persons 65 years of age and older is expected to grow from 24 million presently to 55 million in the year 2030 (HEW 1978, p. 3). HEW (1978, p. 5) states that "judicial decisions requiring that involuntarily committed mentally ill and retarded patients be served in the least restrictive setting could increase spending by billions of dollars."

The CBO estimates that 5.5 to 7.2 million elderly and disabled will require some form of long-term care by 1985 (CBO 1977b, p. 47). They estimate that spending under present law for long-term-care services will rise from $21.3 to $24.1 billion in FY 1977 to $63.7 to $74.5 billion in FY 1985 (CBO 1977b, p. 17).

Any reforms of the present system of long-term care that seek to significantly improve the quality of care or expand eligibility, benefits, and services under public programs (for example, to meet unmet needs, to increase the availability and utilization of noninstitutional care services, to improve equity across the states, to publicly pay for care now privately paid for or provided, or to add case management services) are likely to raise costs higher. Some reforms may increase the efficient utilization of long-term-care services, but they are also likely to raise total costs. Expanded coverage and supply of community care services would lower demand for institutional care and reduce unnecessary and inappropriate utilization of institutional care services, but would probably increase the demand for noninstitutional care and substitute formal care for much informal care. The scale of these shifts has been estimated in crude terms only.

Fragmentation

The present system of long-term care is highly fragmented, both in terms of financing and service delivery. A multitude of programs and agencies at the federal, state, and local levels are involved in long-term care, but no centralized responsibility exists for long-term care at any level. HEW (1978, appendix 10, table 4) lists twenty-six different federal programs that provide resources for persons with long-term-care needs. These programs fund similar services as well as different services, but each has its legislatively mandated eligibility requirements, benefit coverage, regulations for provider participation, administrative structures, and service-delivery mechanisms. They all operate fairly independently at each level of government. Differences between Medicaid, Title XX, and SSI are particularly important as they are largely responsible for the lack of fit between the necessary health, social, and income components of long-term care under the current system (LaVor 1977, pp. 59-63). Programmatic fragmentation has produced a fragmented service-delivery system for long-term care. There are presently a wide variety of disconnected types of facilities, services, and providers that are not tied together in any systematic way. The result is a highly complicated and confused system of long-term care.

Lack of Case Management Functions

It is argued that major reforms are needed in the present system of long-term care because the current system lacks important case management functions. Specifically, no centralized information, referral, and counseling, no centralized comprehensive needs assessment, no central agent for prescribing and designing a comprehensive package of services, and no central agent for pulling together different financial and service resources exist. There is no central rationing agent for allocating limited resources for service delivery and financing among all those with needs for long-term care (particularly for personal social services in community and in-home settings). There is no centralized mechanism for assuring and assisting placement in the most cost-effective care setting, no centralized coordination of service-delivery and funding sources, no centralized patient monitoring and periodic reassessment of needs, and no centralized advocacy for individual patients.

Although professionals argue that case management should be an integral part of any new program for long-term care, case management is especially important for the current system of long-term care. Under the present system, the burden for performing these functions rests primarily with the patients themselves and their families, who are ill-equipped to do so. Under the current system, many programs, services, facilities, providers, and agencies function independently of one another. Program requirements and individual needs are complex. Presently, no one is available to help individuals and families utilize the available resources. Professional experts are needed, it is argued, to help individuals and families deal with the fragmentation and complexity. Expert assistance should improve the appropriate, efficient, and cost-effective utilization of the limited resources available.

Assessment of the Arguments

These arguments for changing the present system have varying degrees of power, but one fact emerges clearly: no one change can address all of the problems identified. The aims of these arguments, seen collectively, are a mélange of contradictions: to broaden the eligibility pool, to control costs and expenditures, to improve quality, to treat all regions and persons equally, and to simplify organization while elaborating service options.

The arguments about unmet needs are only moderately secure because no firm criteria have been developed with which to measure need. Although the evidence about some need is strong, it is not at all clear how severe the needs are or which needs should necessarily be met by public action. Some needs have a strong claim for action only for persons who lack any family resources at all or for persons living in areas with minimal services. The data do not discriminate along these lines.

The argument about family burdens is strong, but action would call for greatly enlarged public responsibility and expenditure and the justification for so large a transfer from private family to public resources has not been developed.

Other problems might be satisfied by structural changes, but the political costs may be higher than the financial costs. The biases to institutional care could be rectified by altering regulatory and financial incentives, the aim being to assure that persons with need have even-handed access to all services in any program finally adopted.

The fragmentation among services and geographic inequity involves maldistribution in one form or another, since some persons benefit from the present system and others do not. The evidence for this aspect is mainly descriptive or based on the assumption that a multiplicity of programs necessarily means fragmentation. Such conclusions would be warranted if there were strong evidence that boundaries between eligible populations and service providers are blurred, duplicative, or discontinuous, but the quantitative evidence is not strong nationally.

Geographic maldistribution relies heavily on a belief, rather than objective evidence, that horizontal equalization is necessary for equity sufficient for public satisfaction. If true, the need could be met by increased appropriations to bring low-service areas up to a higher level or by a reallocation of federal resources from high- to low-resource areas or states (as was the case in Title XX distribution).

Arguments about low quality of care are supported by powerful anecdotal and public-hearing testimony, although strong evaluative data are lacking about the personal damage that results. For example, it is not clear whether the same standards are appropriate for rural as for urban conditions. The extensiveness of neglect and abuse in the target population compared with the proportion adequately cared for is not well documented, and there are no good ways to weigh, for example, social isolation with good care against satisfying social involvement with poor-to-bad physical environments—so that only an ideal state exists for measurement. The criteria are not good with which to judge the seriousness of various deficiencies or failure to achieve the ideal state. Separating the (relatively) good from the ideal is still difficult.

Practically, improving quality of care depends on technical and organizational methods to either motivate or to control innumerable providers and millions of individuals and their family members. If effective controls or motivating techniques are utilized, the result should be an insignificant incidence of low-quality care. However, the absence of effective controls should result in widespread low quality. If controls exist that could improve the quality of care, and they are not being used, it may be because the implementation of these controls would increase the administrative costs and the bureaucratic control over providers, factors which would not necessarily increase service volume or accessibility.

The accumulated evidence for change produces a strong belief that *something* needs altering. But, on closer analysis, few clues powerfully demand any one type of approach—except for the case to expand public expenditures because the burden on families is ultimately disastrous or the case to retain the system because access to service alternatives is not dangerously biased. For the rest, alternative arrangements could incorporate changes that satisfy one or the other demand either by restructuring the long-term-care system materially, with attendant political if not fiscal perturbation, or by increasing public regulatory control and increasing administrative rather than service expenditures.

Previous Analyses of Major Options

The major studies noted earlier also analyzed certain options for reform. These analyses, however, did not attempt a systematic comparison of the major options, one against the other, using a common framework or set of criteria. Since duplicating the efforts made by others would be unwise, the following summary of their conclusions is only noted here. (Details are in the appendix.)

Insurance for Long-Term Care

Insurance for long-term care in national health insurance legislation is concluded to be undesirable by Joe and Meltzer (1976) and Pollak (1974) on the grounds that current and proposed legislation for health insurance is primarily institutionally focused and that, if noninstitutional services are included, replacement of informal care by formal agencies would be difficult to control. However, separate insurance for long-term care outside of national health insurance is also considered by the CBO (1977), Correia (1976), Pollak (1974), and HEW (1974). Generally, these analysts conclude that a better balance between institutional and noninstitutional services might result, but the costs would be very high, although they cannot be accurately estimated. An open-ended federal/state matching program for long-term care is considered by Pollak (1974) and HEW (1974) to be very similar to insurance for long-term conditions with the exception that administration would be transferred from the federal government to the state governments. The conclusions are similar to those for insurance except that, in addition, much more geographic diversity would be expected.

Closed-Ended Federal Grants to States

The option of federal grants is anlayzed by all except Joe and Meltzer (1976). Although evidence to support the argument is sparse, these analysts generally agree that such a program might result in a more equitable geographical distribution of federal funds. The division in financing between health and social services would be reduced; state flexibility to package services for individual needs would be improved; dollars would be redistributed among the states; and gaps would be likely to arise in entitlement in various jurisdictions. Pollak (1974) considers that this option is inappropriate, except as a complement to an interim Medicaid program. HEW (1976) chose this option, but HEW (1978) thought that such a program would only be appropriate in conjunction with a national health insurance program that offered significant fiscal relief to states for acute care.

Specialized Funding

A wide variety of specialized options have been proposed to provide funding differentiated by site of delivery or by type of cost to be met. These are analyzed by Joe and Meltzer (1976), Correia (1976), and by HEW (1974, 1978). Since innumerable variations exist for such specialized funding, only main themes are noted here. One type would provide one source of funding for institutional care with federal/state matching and an open-ended federal share. A separate program for community and in-home services, although also matched, would be administered by states with closed-ended federal funding. A different form of separate funding is one in which all medical costs would be covered by a form of national health insurance, whereas other living and social-support costs would be defrayed by some combination of individual payment and independent social-welfare programs.

In general, the analysts seem to consider that these divisions in program funding have certain advantages that might be difficult to carry out. The first type, for example, would, at a minimum, underwrite the maintenance of two systems: one for institutional care and one for noninstitutional care, each with its own delivery and financing system. However, the response of state governments to any set of programs of this nature would be difficult to predict; it is likely, however, that states would utilize those programs that are most financially beneficial. One problem that could arise is that limiting the transfer of funding from state to federal sources would be difficult. However, while the separation of program funding by site or by cost function (medicine or social welfare) involves the redistribution of much of the long-term-care cost burden to welfare programs or to the states, it may involve a more effective accounting of actual costs that are appropriate for each type of funding source.

Cash Payments and Vouchers to Individuals

Pollak (1974) and Correia (1976) consider the cashing-out option to be very costly, although they differ about the administrative difficulties that would be entailed. Only Pollak considers vouchers but comes to no strong conclusion about their use.

Local Long-Term-Care Organizations

Correia (1976) and HEW (1976, 1978) considered this option. The organizations would have primary responsibility for assessment, planning, coordination, and control of the flow of resources to direct providers. The analysts appear to conclude that, despite the advantages in flexibility and individual case packaging that might result, significant disadvantages are present: There is an unwarranted assumption that valid assessment techniques are available, development would be very uneven by jurisdiction (producing gaps in services), and the operation would be very costly.

Framework for Comparative Analysis
of Six Options

A new analysis is worthwhile only if it significantly improves understanding of the subject. Within the limitations noted here, the analysis of options in this chapter differs from its predecessors in three ways:

1. It examines each of the six options against a common set of criteria (see p. 6) a comparison that may clarify how any one option could correct system defects when measured against the probable results of the other options.
2. It examines what can be expected to result if any one option is adopted, as well as what goals that option promises to achieve.
3. It considers the long-term-care field as a system of largely independent elements, the functioning of which could be improved by a better-designed federal policy.

Limitations in Analysis

Analytic efforts in the past have been circumscribed by several limiting factors that affect the current effort. Although much more is known now than before, these limitations warn us that conclusions should be treated as reasonable best estimates, given the state of knowledge and of the art, not as solidly proven facts. The major limitations are summarized in the next sections.

Nature of the Problem

Long-term-care difficulties are produced in part by the evolution of a new situation in American society—the survival of large numbers of severely disabled persons at a time when the economy draws most able-bodied adults, including wives, into paid employment, which diminishes the family-care resources. Imperfections in the organization and funding of long-term programs in both health and welfare are embedded in, and may result in part from, difficulty in controlling these two basic social developments. Attempts to control and structure expenditures more effectively are offset against changing pressures that are not well predicted. At a minimum, control of costs and improved equity are contending goals.

Data Limitations

Much now is known about populations-at-risk and about the variables that affect their dependency. But only at the extremes of very mild or very severe disablement do data-array patients clearly fit along any continuum of care or service need. Large gray areas obscure the extent to which some services might substitute for others; for example, home care for nursing home care. Estimates of inappropriate placement in institutions are, in part, artificial constructs based on expert judgments about a physical condition but do not take into account social constraints such as lack of family-support back-up, low income, or patient mobility limitation on the use of available services. Perhaps one-third of cases with like disability are found equally in nursing institutions and at home.

Excellent assessment instruments have been developed and standard-ized, but they are costly to apply widely and little is known about how these assessments translate into the actual procurement of recommended service packages.

The costing of alternative approaches is hampered by differences in the way data are reported by different providers: for example, ratios of per-sonnel used in relation to population served are reported differently by nursing homes, by home health agencies, and by home care agencies so that comparative costing is crude.

Little is firmly known whether home care replaces or only delays admis-sion to an institution.

Unclear Categories

Provider agencies in long-term care tend to be small and numerous, com-pared, for example, to hospitals. Their classification varies state by state despite progress toward federal standardization. No clear boundary demar-cation exists between many of the providers and few people agree about what the boundaries should be or how the categories should be defined. At-tempts at definition have, in their turn, produced a proliferation of specialties—for example, home health aides, homemakers, chore workers, home helps, mobility aides, and so forth, whose functions may be overlap-ping. Even among the options advanced for improving the situation, substantial overlap can be found in the way insurance or disability allowances are perceived, or in the way case management or a single long-term agency is defined.

System Interactions

A minimum foundation has been laid in data to trace the functioning of formal health-and-welfare-agency interactions in meeting the needs of the long-term patient. But, the dominant care component—the informal net-work of family and friends—is very little understood except in the most general terms. The flow between the informal and formal systems of care, what governs the movement to and fro, and what is best performed by each segment for what types of patients are only now beginning to be studied, but the study itself is affected by many subjective judgments.

Among the components of the formal care system, some data are beginning to emerge. The flow between acute-care and long-term medical or health agencies and the concomitant flow between health-financed agencies and agencies financed by welfare sources, however, is determined more by conflicting public policies than by the requirements of a rationally designed system. Data can be used to estimate reasonably what the effect of any one policy is likely to be on the functioning of the formal care system, but it cannot help choose among contradictory public policies.

These limitations, however, should not discourage analysis of the long-term-care sector but rather serve to stimulate and improve the quality of the data available.

References

Branch, L. 1978. *Boston Elders*. Cambridge, Mass.: Joint Center for Urban Studies.

Commission on Chronic Illness. 1956. *Care for the Long-Term Patient*. Cambridge, Mass.: Harvard University Press, pp. 19-20.

Congressional Budget Office (CBO). 1977a. "Long-Term Care for the Elderly and Disabled." (February):16-17.

———. 1977b. "Long-Term Care: Actuarial Cost Estimates." (August): table 7, p. 27.

Correia, E. 1976. "National Health Insurance, Welfare Reform, and the Disabled: Issues in Program Reform." Prepared for Office of the Assistant Secretary for Planning and Evaluation, U.S. Department of Health, Education and Welfare, Washington, D.C., August.

Eggert, G., et al. 1977. "Caring for the Patient with Long-Term Disability." *Geriatrics* 32, no. 10 (October):3-20.

Gibson, R.M., and Fisher, C.R. 1978. "National Health Expenditures, Fiscal Year 1977," *Social Security Bulletin* (July):3-20.

Gurland, B. 1978. *Dependency Among the Elderly in New York*. New York Community Council of Greater New York.

Joe, T. and Meltzer, J. 1976. "Policies and Strategies for Long-Term Care." San Francisco: Health Policy Program, University of California, May 14.

Klerman, L. 1978. "A Follow-up Study of Children Handicapped at Birth." Waltham, Mass.: Brandeis University, Levinson Policy Institute.

LaVor, Judith. 1977. "Long-Term Care: A Challenge to Service Systems," Office of the Assistant Secretary for Planning and Evaluation, U.S. Department of Health, Education and Welfare. Washington, D.C., April.

Mendelson, M. 1974. *Tender Loving Greed*. New York: Alfred A. Knopf.

Pollak, W. 1974. "Federal Long-Term Care Strategy: Options and Analysis," The Urban Institute, 17 October 1973, revised 25 February 1974.

U.S. Department of Health, Education and Welfare (HEW), Office of the Secretary. 1974. "Program Design Choices For Long-Term Care Legislative Initiative—Decision Memorandum." Washington, D.C., August.

_____ . Office of the Secretary, 1976. "Long-Term Care Services Legislative Proposal." Washington, D.C., October 19.

_____ . Office of the Secretary. 1978. "Memorandum for July 14, 1978, Briefing, Major Initiative: Long-Term Care/Community Services." Washington, D.C., p. 3 and appendix 10, table 1.

_____ . National Center for Health Statistics. 1979. *The National Nursing Home Survey: 1977 Summary for the United States* Washington, D.C., July.

Part II
Options for Financing
Long-Term Care

Three distinct options for financing long-term care are discussed in part II. They are the bloc grant, a national compulsory long-term-care-insurance program, and a federal disability allowance voucher program. All of these proposals are concerned with ways of meeting long-term-care needs, yet also with assuring efficient expenditures of funds.

Robert Hudson in chapter 3 examines the concept of a bloc grant and reviews recent experience with some bloc grant programs. He applies lessons learned to what might occur under a bloc grant for long-term. In Hudson's assessment, the bloc grant might be a successful mechanism for limiting the expenditure of funds in long-term care, but its impact on meeting human needs may be less than positive. Hudson's main point seems to be that the state-level political process engendered by the need to allocate limited and fixed resources to a variety of long-term-care purposes could reduce alternatives and constrain the development of new services. Success of any bloc grant approach would be highly dependent on continued federal involvement in enforcing legislative and regulatory provisions of the bloc grant legislation. He notes that perhaps the only financial "carrot" large enough to induce states to accept a bloc grant would be a national health insurance program that relieved the states of Medicaid.

Christine Bishop in chapter 4 presents a convincing case that the private insurance industry cannot offer comprehensive policies insuring against the risk of long-term care disabilities. Bishop points out the significance of the insurance problems of adverse selection and moral hazard for long-term care and identifies some unique problem factors resulting from the nature of long-term-care needs and the services required to meet them. Among these factors are definitions of benefits and the relationship of noncompensated family services to the benefit structure. Bishop concludes that the only way to overcome these problems is through a national compulsory program where individuals insure themselves early in life for the increasing probability of becoming disabled as they grow older. Bishop proposes that efficiency in allocating resources be built on the elements of consumer choice and copayment. She describes how this approach would be as adaptable to the poor as to the rich. Despite the strong tilt toward consumer control, a large federal role is maintained, not only in the financing of the system but also in personal needs assessment, rate regulation, and quality control.

Gruenberg and Pillemer in chapter 5 focus their analysis on a disability allowance approach. While this approach has some of the features of the insurance option in that it prescribes the covered benefits, it is structured so as to be close to a cash-based system. Comparisons to a cash program are presented throughout the chapter. To avoid some of the economic and political problems usually associated with assistance-type programs, the authors describe a program that is capable of differentiating individuals by degree of need, family status, and income. While constraining the eligibility and payment level, considerable consumer sovereignty remains. In this discussion they briefly allude to the preponderance of cash programs in Western European countries. These countries have been able to overcome the reluctance of public officials to provide cash. By not including an income and assets test in their proposals, Gruenberg and Pillemer may have developed a politically acceptable compromise.

All three of these options maintain a large role for the federal government in financing these programs and insuring that they are effective and efficient in meeting human needs. There apears to be no way to release the federal government from its responsibility in financing long-term-care problems.

Other common themes appear, but particularly in the insurance and disability allowance options, the issues of assessments, type and scope of benefits, and role of the informal caregiver network are most visible. These issues and some proposed answers will reappear in Part III when the organizational options are presented.

3

Restructuring Federal/State Relations in Long-Term Care: The Bloc Grant Alternative

Robert B. Hudson

A bloc grant to the states for long-term-care purposes is one potential option for addressing the fragmented, uneven, and extremely costly long-term-care "system" now in place. Among other things, it is argued a long-term-care bloc grant would allow for greater control and coordination of service delivery and could do so at a level of government—the state level—that is closer to the problem and could thus be more responsive in dealing with it. As currently envisaged, federal financial participation would be capped near present levels, with the designated agencies in the states receiving a formula-based bloc grant for long-term-care purposes. Unlike the present system under Medicaid—the principal source of public long-term-care funds—states would not automatically be reimbursed for a fixed percentage of all costs they incur. This feature capping federal funding, unless the level is exceptionally generous, will lead to both absolute and relative cost increases for state long-term-care programs. Indirect relief would be forthcoming to the states if proposals to nationalize financing of acute care services for the aged, poor, and working poor materialize in the early 1980s.

The first part of this chapter reviews arguments, both pro and con, about the feasibility and utility of a formula-based, multipurpose- (bloc) grant system. The latter part of this chapter applies these arguments to the long-term-care policy area and sets them against particular long-term-care policy concerns: distribution of cost, effects on consumers and providers, locus of program control, and political barriers to implementation of such a program. In each of these areas, major problems arise concerning both the feasibility and desirability of pursuing the bloc-grant option in long-term care. Conceptually, the bloc grant alternative brings with it a number of programmatic benefits, but many of these, it is argued, may vanish in practice. A bloc grant's working in accordance with the underlying programmatic intent rests on a number of assumptions about the incentives and agendas of involved parties, the structure or setting in which those agendas are played out, and the particulars of the policy area itself. In the case of long-term care, there is good reason to suspect that several of the requisite assumptions cannot be made or relied on.

The Bloc Grant Mechanism

The major dimension along which grants-in-aid are ranged is one delineating both scope of programmatic activity and discretion allowed of state officials. Three generic types of grants are conventionally placed among this dimension: (1) categorical (narrow in scope, limited discretion); (2) bloc (broader in scope, allowing more discretion); and (3) revenue sharing (very broad in scope, nearly unlimited discretion). Through the late 1960s, most grants-in-aid were of the categorical kind, specifying that federal funds be spent for specifically designated purposes (sewer construction, library services, lead-paint-poisoning prevention) in accordance with restrictive legislative and regulative provisions. The growth in the number of these grants during the 1960s created numerous vertical (federal/state) programmatic authorities that in turn created major problems or coordination and control at the state level. State governors and planning officials were particularly disturbed by the cumulative consequences of these grants, arguing that too many upward lines of authority made it increasingly difficult to manage programs at the state level.[1] The vertical ties inherent in this grant mechanism were captured nicely in Terry Sanford's phrase, "picket-fence federalism."[2]

As a means of assisting state officials (and under the New Federalism, cutting back the role of federal officials), moves began in the late 1960s to consolidate related functions and to provide greater latitude to state officials. The general need for such changes was sounded in the Intergovernmental Cooperation Act of 1968, and the first major piece of bloc grant legislation embodying these concerns came in the Partnership for Health Act of 1967. Since then the bloc grant concept has been reflected in the comprehensive employment, community development, and social services (Title XX) legislation. In each of these cases, related functions under earlier legislation have been collapsed under one authority, and the role of federal officials in the setting of programmatic priorities and the specification of appropriate implementation mechanisms has been curtailed. Areas of policy intent are set forth, but the guiding language is usually confined to overall legislative goals rather than specific programmatic objectives.

Farther along this grants-in-aid continuum are special- and general-revenue sharing. The demarcation point between bloc grants and special-revenue sharing is murky, with the latter type differing in its requiring either a very minor or no state financial participation. A sum of federal funds is turned over to the states for broad purposes. Such a proposal was put forth for the social services, but the Title XX legislation—mandating 25 percent state effort, goal statements, and procedural requirements—emerged in its place because of concerns of a coalition of social-welfare professionals and providers that there be some legislative language confining the program and protecting their interests. General revenue sharing—as embodied in current law—requires no financial participation of states and localities, and the funds can be used for any of eight encompassing policy areas. While this legislation has provided considerable fiscal relief to subnational jurisdictions, it has been widely criticized on grounds that it is used largely for highly visible "bricks-and-mortar" projects and that it allows the most highly organized (and better-off) policy interests unrestricted opportunity to use their disproportionate political muscle. This last argument has also been voiced in opposition to the bloc grant and special-revenue approaches and will be raised here in reference to the long-term-care bloc-grant option.

The Case for Bloc Grants

The arguments in favor of utilizing the bloc grant approach as a means of financing the administering of domestic policy through the federal system can be placed under five headings as follows.

Improving Program Coordination Near the Point of Delivery. The bloc-grant approach—by grouping existing programs under a single legislative and administrative structure—greatly increases the possibilities that related functions could be addressed in a more coordinated fashion. The existence of categorical programs—large in number, narrow in scope, and fragmented in operation—creates a situation in which related functions are carried out in relatively autonomous policy spheres. The result, as reported endlessly in recent years, has often been a pattern in which related efforts are duplicated, and clients with similar needs are unevenly served. By grouping functions and clients under singular and broad program coverage, a bloc grant increases both service efficiency and equity. Resources can be developed or pooled through a single planning process, administrators and providers are forced to generate service modalities that are complementary and reinforcing rather than inconsistent and redundant, and clients (or case managers) are able to draw from a broad array of services in putting together appropriate service packages. There may be varying levels of hierarchical authority directing these efforts and mobilizing the requisite resources, but the bloc grant's at least nominally making program domain broader and more inclusive and represents an important first step in overcoming the "balkanization" that usually characterizes the domestic grant-in-aid terrain.

Eliminating Excessive Decision-Making Junctures between Federal and State Governments. While broadening the scope for decision making at the state level, the bloc grant also reduces the volume and nature of federal officials' activities in the implementation of federal policy. Within broad parameters, the types and relative amounts of different services to be offered and the manner in which that mix should be delivered becomes very much a state-level choice. This choice my have several advantages. First, a major problem revealed in a variety of implementation studies is hereby addressed—that being the number of decision makers and decision-making junctures involved in the implementation process. It is well recognized that a certain amount of "slippage" occurs—by virtue of miscommunications, inability to comply, unwillingness to comply—as policies wend their way from enactment to the point of final delivery. The bloc grant, by greatly reducing the role of central- and regional-office federal officials, largely eliminates the role of actors who, under other circumstances, have been heavily involved in the transmission process between legislative enactment and services delivery.

Second and more substantively, this reduced role for federal officials allows states to adapt the broad guidelines of federal policy to their needs without the federal bureaucratic involvement that the states often see as interference and misdirected involvement. A third presumed advantage is the reduced effort directed toward formal compliance of federal administrative directives. Both state and delivery agencies complain of the volumes of paperwork and other energy that are consumed in federal reporting mechanisms and contend that these requirements often neither guide their actions nor assure meaningful compliance.

Fostering Institution Building at the State Level. An important consequence of the changes brought by the bloc grant is that they may contribute to institution building at the state level. The broadened purpose and scope inherent in the bloc grant and the concomitant reduction in the federal role combine to give greater latitude and control to state-level actors. More important yet is that, within the state, control gravitates to general-purpose governments rather than to special-purpose ones and to generalist officials rather than to program officials. The greatest complaint state governors, planners, and budget officials have had with categorical grants was that the lines of authority were primarily between corresponding program officials in the federal, regional, state, and substate offices charged with program administration. Federal funds have become an increasing part of state budgets, and so long as they came through the categorical mechanism (whether on a formula or project basis), "staff" officials had minimal control over the purposes and distribution of those funds. Inherent in the logic of bloc grants is the clear potential to redraw these lines of authority, giving the governor and his or her office a much greater voice in program planning and implementation.

The heightened role given these officials can serve to greatly strengthen the policy performance of state-level actors. They are given both the responsibility to assure that policy intent is followed during the implementation process and the command over resources associated with the policy—primarily authority and funding. Combined with the other formal and informal powers of their offices, the governor and his or her staff are now well positioned to provide program direction in keeping with the strictures of a conventional management-control approach to administration. With these records in hand, the governor et al. possess the wherewithal to oversee the development of comprehensive and coordinated program initiative in the substantive area at hand. Proximate responsibility will still, of course, lie with line officials directly charged with implementation, but their actions are now guided by hierarchical officials at the state level who are, in turn, accountable to an electorate in the jurisdiction where implementation is taking place.

Allowing Greater Citizen Input by Virtue of Having Decision Making Located "Closer to the People." Choice-making and implementation under a bloc grant may be more democratic and responsive to citizen needs than in the narrower, federally involved categorical-grant system. A first reason for this contention was alluded to just previously: elected state leadership is vested with critical decision-making authority regarding the policy's administration within the state, and disagreement with that process can be sounded through the conventional participatory devices of voting, lobbying, letter-writing, and so forth. Under the categorical-grant system, vertical domains are tight and often impenetrable (even governors complained), and decisions were made by career officials in Washington.

A second factor centers on provisions that are usually (but not always) included in bloc-grant legislation. Procedures to ensure citizen or consumer participation in the implementation process are found in the Title XX, Health Planning and Resources Development, and other legislation. Common provisions call for citizen participation in advisory committees, the holding of public hearings on state plans, and designated time periods in which citizen and other groups may comment on proposed actions. Data on the effectiveness of these mechanisms remain sketchy, but the requirement for input is there even if its impact is unclear.

A third reason for expecting greater responsiveness and participation under the bloc-grant concept centers on the breadth of the grants and the locus of decision making being closer to the people at the state level than it is at the national level. Within the state planning process, the wide range of professionals, providers, and clients are able (depending in part on the procedural stipulations of the grant program in question) to work on the development of programs suited to the perceived service needs within the state. Where differences arise, these people are then able to enter a process of negotiation and bargaining and are presumably able to reach compromises that reflect a reasonable balance of service needs in the state. While there clearly may be pitfalls in this process, the parties involved in it can be expected to have greater familiarity with the array of needs and resources within the state than might be found at the federal level.

Recognizing Variations in the Program Needs and Structural Make-up of the States. Finally, the bloc grant brings with it greater programmatic flexibility than the categorical grant. Whatever merit the argument that the states may serve as "laboratories" for experimentation and innovation may have, bloc grants allow for a more reasonable empirical test than do more restrictive grant-in-aid options. Under the bloc grant system, greater latitude is provided to the states in such decisions as the locus and organization of substate planning and delivery mechanisms, ways of packaging service functions and client populations, and determining appropriate ways to evaluate service inputs and client outcomes.

Bloc grants are also better able to accommodate cross-state variations relevant to service priorities and delivery. These variations along any number of demographic, economic, and political dimensions are, of course, very considerable. Particularly important is the ratio of service resources to service needs, and variations here may require quite different implementation approaches. Under these circumstances, greater flexibility inherent in the bloc-grant approach is a virtue.

By allowing some greater latitude for experimentation, bloc grants may be a most appropriate programmatic response in those substantive policy areas where the knowledge base is weak. The knowledge problem remains severe in many aspects of health care and social services.[3] In part, the question is: What do given policies propose to optimize (self-support, independent living, deinstitutionalization, cost-efficiencies, and so on)? But even where agreement can be reached about these value questions, information about what intervention strategies and techniques yield particular client outcomes is usually sketchy and/or in need of improved validity and reliability. Under these circumstances, a good case can be made for allowing multiple modes of service intervention, and the flexibility associated with the bloc-grant approach may be well suited to fostering multiple approaches.

The Case against Bloc Grants

The problems that potentially arise—and have arisen—under the bloc grant alternative result from the way the implementation process is structured and how that imperfect process allows relevant actors to play out particular agendas of their own. The bloc grant concept weakens the authority of the agency charged with overseeing policy implementation (1) by reducing its legislative authority or "protection" and (2) by increasing the role of other agencies, groups, and clients who are unevenly positioned for influencing the decision-making process. In short, the bloc grant approach combines two models of implementation—the management control approach and the pluralist or market approach—and in so doing vitiates some of the advantages inherent in each of them when taken separately. The consequences of this mixing will be visible in critical stages of the implementation process, most notably in service choice and program accountability.

The Role and Resources of the
Designated State Agency

At first glance, it would appear that whatever agency is designated to administer a new bloc grant program is strengthened almost by definition. Its scope of activity, responsibilities, and funding are expanded as existing authorities are folded under its aegis or new authority is created. It is free of detailed mandates emanating from the federal level while being given programmatic responsibility for the use of federal funds.

The major problems that may arise for the designated state agency (DSA) under these circumstances are primarily bureaucratic and organizational. First, the withdrawal of strict federal regulations, while seemingly freeing the DSA to pursue its own course of action, also removes what may be considered either a source of support of a "scapegoat" for the actions the DSA takes. Under the categorical system, the DSA is able to refer benefit-seeking clients, contract-demanding providers, and cost-conscious budget officials to federal requirements that precluded the DSA from making major moves to satisfy any of them. With the federal involvement or excuse largely missing, the DSA is placed in a position of having to defend its action or nonaction on substantive or other grounds that it devised itself.

Second, the withdrawn federal support may not be replaced by support from officials at the state level. As indicated earlier, it is argued that the bloc-grant approach enables generalist officials—governors, planners, budget officials—to make the policy more of their own and direct it in ways of their own choosing. However, depending on the policy in question, these officials may wish to have little to do with it, or may bring to the program institutional concerns of their own that may be seen as dysfunctional for the manifest purposes of the program. The imperatives of the statewide gubernatorial office, particularly during fiscally difficult times as in the early 1970s and in the present period, call for avoiding the need to generate new state revenues through taxes. Bloc grants have proved useful for hardpressed governors (and mayors) in times of financial stress. Under Title IV-A (a predecessor to Title XX), Comprehensive Employment and Training Act (CETA), Economic Development Act (EDA), and community-development bloc grant programs, much documentation shows that federal funds have been heavily used for "substitutive" rather than "additive" purposes. Being legally, electorally, and symbolically charged with overall leadership in the states, governors may often be more responsive to tax-paying than service-demanding groups. This aspect is particularly true in health-and-welfare programs for disadvantaged groups. These cost concerns of the state's executive leadership often leave the DSA alone and underfunded in meeting its administrative and oversight functions in the implementation process.

Where a bloc grant is imposed on a policy and bureaucratic system that was previously the province of multiple state agencies operating under separate categorical grants, the DSA will also find itself facing the resistance of these heretofore autonomous units. Where these agencies and functions are folded into the DSA, it will weaken the sense of purpose and cohesion necessary for an agency to develop; where some of these agencies remain in existence outside of the DSA, it will make for bureaucratic skirmishing, which can only be debilitating for DSA. As documented by numerous analysts of government reorganization, the presumed advantages of merging functions and shaking up established routine may be lost in the way of the jealousy and turf battles that such consolidation inevitably produces (Seidman 1975).

A third source of political support for the DSA often found under the narrow and hierarchical categorical-grant system—service providers and clients—may become significantly more fractionalized and diffused under the bloc grant system. The broader coverage of the bloc grant brings under the same policy a number of groups with different, competing, and perhaps inconsistent policy interests. Under these circumstances, the close symbiotic relations found among public agencies, legislative committees, and private interests are expanded into a much looser confederation in which major differences may exist. As a matter of public policy, breaking up the tight alliances found under the categorical-grant system is often a good thing, but the weight of making the broader bloc-grant system work falls to the DSA. The mutual exchange of support that may mark the categorical-grant system can be transformed into a situation in which service and client clusterings now make what the DSA must consider excessive demands on its limited resources. The same problem may be true for individual legislators and legislative committees; whereas formerly they had provided support for the discrete program functions, they now too make demands in a larger and more competitive program environment nominally controlled by the DSA.

The cumulative effect of the legislative parameters and multiple agendas at work under the bloc grant system is to put the DSA in a situation where a great imbalance may occur between demand and support. Legal protection is withdrawn and hierarchical support is not forthcoming at the same time that a higher volume of multiple demands is being made on the agency. Where an extreme imbalance exists, the DSA might well find itself in a state referred to by Eisenstadt (1959) as "debureaucratization," a state in which the agency loses virtually all of its autonomy and latitude and is moved according to the balance of outside forces pressing on it. While debureaucratization is an extreme state, an agency's ability to decide its own fate and that of the program it administers is very much dependent on the demand/support balance. Where demands exceed support, a natural inclination of a DSA would be an insular one—that is, drawing back into a bureaucratic "shell" and following a "least-risk" strategy. In the absence of some overwhelming crisis, this strategy then largely leaves the program either static and inflexible or open to changes dictated by the vagaries of outside pressures.

The Roles and Resources of Outside
Interested Parties

While legislative provisions of different bloc grants differ, implicit market (economics) or pluralist (political science) assumptions are usually made concerning the implementation process. Formal participation or involvement by clients and other actors germane to the policy's implementation is established through boards, committees, and public meetings. Informal participation takes place through the ongoing process of consultation and interaction between the DSA and outside actors. In these ways, the hierarchical authority of the DSA (and state officials above the DSA) is conditioned and circumscribed. In mixing the management-control and market models, the result is a situation in which the DSA, depending on its resources as discussed previously, may be little more than "first among equals." The problems confronting the leadership function of the DSA were just reviewed; the issue here is how "equal" are the outside parties that join the implementation process.

For a market or pluralist system to function appropriately, whether in policy implementation or more generally, certain assumptions must be met. Among the principal assumptions are the following: the implementation arena is open to all interested parties; groups are able to organize around salient policy interests; the differential strength of these groups is an accurate reflection of the overall balance of preferences; a sufficient number of organized groups exist so that no one of them may become dominant;

the choices or decisions made during the implementation process result from negotiations and compromises made by the interested groups; and the policy outputs of the implementation process reflect the balance of competing interests. Where these requisites are met, much can be said for the market approach in that implementation decisions are made through what amounts to a well-functioning democratic process. And, because in the present context, all of this is taking place in relatively small jurisdictions as the states, it is frequently argued and assumed that these assumptions may be valid.

The problems here result when, as is often the case, the assumptions are not met. Critics argue and experience often shows that the process is not open to all persons, organized interests vary greatly in power and access, their strength does not accurately reflect the distribution and intensity of policy-related needs, relatively strong groups may choose to cooperate (in essence, a form of collusion) rather than compete, and the implementation outputs are skewed in favor of these groups.

On the question of which individuals and interests are able to organize and press their demands, there can be no doubt that persons who are poor, dependent, and isolated will be less involved in policy implementation than other groups, just as is the case with broader political participation. This problem is exacerbated by the pattern of advocacy-based organization frequently corresponding to that of client-based organization—that is, many of the same groups that find organizing themselves difficult also may tend not to have advocates organizing on their behalf. The needs of many individuals do not fit neatly into age, disability, or service cohorts that tend to attract advocates. Insofar as a high probability exists that the needs of these individuals may also be among the most intractable suggests that these persons are doubly disadvantaged. A major psychic reward of altruism is seeing the positive results of one's efforts; for the most disadvantaged groups, such results are the most difficult to bring about.

Advocates and providers who have become either well entrenched under earlier legislation or well positioned enough to influence the implementation of new legislation may be disposed to join forces during implementation negotiations in order to protect "market share" in the face of new and different functions that are being folded into a given bloc grant. Under these circumstances, the actual merits and desirability of what they are providing and whom they are serving is not germane; they will simply work to protect their own service domains and, in so doing, will impede the development of alternative types of services and, perhaps, new groups of clients.

A final dysfunction of the openness of the bloc-grant-implementation process focuses on political considerations. In order to create the impression that a wide variety of parties are being heard and listened to, the DSA will see it in its interest to provide at least token funding for services and clients located throughout the state. The "statewideness" feature found in all federal grants necessitates some of this tokenism, but the particular distribution to given providers and for given sets of clients may, again, very much reflect the organizational strength of these groups and also the constituency interests of state legislators. Where the law is sufficiently open, political concerns of the most blatant kind can be a major factor in how grant funds are distributed.

The discussion thus far in this section has been directed toward setting forth the potential difficulties created by a bloc grant's mixing two implementation models—management control and market.[4] The bloc-grant approach takes from the DSA the resources and incentives to bring strong direction to the program's implementation, while opening up the implementation process to outside forces that may have the ability to move the program and its funds in ways that are not consonant with a rational or impartial assessment of policy-related needs. This section concludes with a brief discussion of the more specific consequences these factors may have for service choices and for program accountability.

Service Choices

Under a bloc-grant system, the states are presumably better able to package services to meet the needs of potential clients because of the loosening of federal restrictions. Because of fiscal constraints and nonprogrammatic agendas of involved parties, a very illusory quality to this presumed advantage of the bloc-grant system can emerge. And, the changes that do take place may be undertaken for the wrong reasons and be directed away from needed services and needy clients.

The amount of change and flexibility to be expected is relatively low because the bloc grant does not come to a neutral environment. Funding levels are likely to be little different than under preceding arrangements, and the policy space created by those funds is already occupied. Whatever the wisdom of the earlier strictures that directed funds into certain areas (and however much they may have originally been resisted), those directives and funds led to the development of selected allocative patterns, and most of them will not be easily changed simply because at a second point in time they are no longer mandatory. The cumulation of these factors—lessened central direction, occupied policy space, and limited amounts of new money—combine to make the bloc grant alternative a conservative one in the temporal sense. The "engine" that might make change is largely removed, and the remaining parts have a vested interest in keeping things as they were.

The changes in service allocations most likely to develop under these circumstances are away from those areas and clients that were politically unpopular, difficult, or unpleasant and not cost-efficient to persons required to make the service available. The political variable is important here; groups that have been targeted and protected by earlier federal legislation are now (depending on the provisions of the particular bloc grant) left to the vagaries of state-level politics. Under these conditions, there is a marked tendency—seen under Title XX, Comprehensive Employment and Training Act (CETA), Elementary and Secondary Education Act (ESEA)—for funds to be allocated less toward needy areas and clients than a literal reading of legislative intent would suggest. Where the law does not have teeth and the provider groups serving the very needy do not have access and influence, these groups may find the volume of services directed toward them diminishing, although for reasons that are essentially symbolic, coverage will not disappear altogether. More pervasive may be providers who have previously served a wide array of clients now changing their service mix away from the hard-core problems—the so-called creaming phenomenon. In the abstract, giving any precise estimate of how much of this might occur is not possible, but where a major legislative safeguard such as means testing were eliminated or "liberalized," one could expect a shift away from low-income and high-disability clients. Political appeal, ease of service delivery, and organizational "profits" (money, prestige, "success") all contribute to this pattern.

More broadly, what this argument highlights is the fallacious element of the contention, used often in conjunction with the bloc-grant alternative, that the states are a more responsive locus at which to have service choices made. Essentially, what this argument does is to confuse democracy with decentralization.[5] While decentralization does place decision making closer to the persons affected by the decisions taken, the more important way of understanding decentralization is to note that the jurisdictions in which decisions are made are thereby made smaller. The consequences of this decentralization, as argued by theorists dating back to James Madison, are that highly organized interests may more easily control the decision-making process and that decision making is controlled less through the formality of law and more through the informality of informal connections and networks. Both of these aspects are seen as resulting in a situation in which "have-not" groups remain so as established groups are able to continue long-standing domination. As stated in a broader context by Schattschneider (1960), "the problem in the pluralist [market] heaven is that the choir sings with a decidedly upper-class accent." The argument continues that the have-not groups fare better when the "scope of conflict is expanded," which in the present context, would suggest that the devolution of program control from the federal to the state level does not auger well for disadvantaged groups.

Program Accountability

A second set of programmatic concerns generated by the bloc grant alternative centers on program accountability. Under the management-control approach to implementation associated with categorical grants, accountability is upward—to hierarchical officials and the provisions of law and regulation. Under the bloc grant system, responsibility for accountability lies with the DSA that is also administering the program with generalist leadership at the state level. Federal regulations under the bloc grant system may be limited only to complying with overall program goals and selected procedures to be followed in the determination of services to be developed. Apart from questions of enforcement (to be considered momentarily) these differences have substantive consequences. Under the categorical/management-control approach, accountability is principally a matter of ascertaining levels of compliance with legislative requirements and the effectiveness of implemented services. Accountability revolves around determining what was done and whether it made any difference. Under the bloc-grant system, depending on its openness, the accountability questions most relevant to federal officials center more on procedures and responsiveness. Was the process an open one and did the resulting services reflect the input of those parties who availed themselves of the opportunity to participate? Issues germane to program operation are now more the responsibility of state-level actors.

An issue at the state level concerns where responsibility for program operation will be lodged. Certainly, the DSA will be charged with monitoring and assessing the performance of providers funded under its auspices. Because of the support/demand imbalance the DSA may be confronted with and the posture it may assume as a result, questioning how strong a stance it will be willing and able to take in enforcing its own rules is important. The DSA may variously choose to see its role as a dispenser of benefits, a referee in the competition for funds, a generator of new service approaches, or a protector of the most disadvantaged persons potentially affected by its programs. How the DSA chooses to define its role will have differential consequences for program enforcement. Of equal concern is which of these roles the DSA may be able to consider organizationally prudent to assume given the environment in which it may be operating. The DSA will already have consumed some amount of goodwill in deciding whom and what to fund and not fund. To then go about the yet more enervating task of enforcing compliance may well appear as an unwise course of action.

Forceful leadership and the backing of hierarchical state officials can serve to reduce these concerns by providing important resources to the DSA, but these ingredients cannot be expected to exist in all of the fifty jurisdictions charged with overseeing bloc grant implementation. The existence of state executive and program leadership, moreover, can be expected to move in tandem. Governors concerned with program performance will make a point of appointing agency heads who share that concern and have demonstrated ability to be effective in such a task.

Acknowledging the electoral idiosyncracies that might establish effective leaders, the incentive structure of electoral politics mitigates against overriding concern with program enforcement. In the literature on policy implementation, the observation that minimal payoffs are available for presidents, governors, and majors who devote major energies to how policies are implemented has become axiomatic. The implementation process is long in time, low in visibility, and usually has low political currency. As for legislators, the case against concern with implementation is made more strongly yet; their role is simply not associated with implementation concerns unless a particular scandal or bit of political casework is involved that they can engage in to bring media or constituent attention. Implementation does not find a place on a legislative agenda that, in Mayhew's (1974) words, is composed of concern with credit claiming, advertising, and garnering particularistic benefits for the folks back home. This absence of concern with implementation associated with elected officials—and especially rectifying errant behavior as required in rendering programs accountable—leaves the DSA to its own devices, which may be few.

A final source of accountability under the bloc grant system would lie in the market aspect of bloc grants' functioning in accordance with the model's theoretical advantages. Thus, if relatively pure competition existed among providers—the same services being offered in the same geographical location to the same persons—consumer choice would serve as the accountability mechanism. Persons dissatisfied with what was being offered by a given provider could "shop around" and gravitate to the provider who was performing in a manner most consonant with the consumers' needs and expectations. However, well-known problems exist with this system that, if it worked appropriately, this system would be preferable to all other alternatives. Lack of consumer information and collusion among supposedly competing providers are among the most notable. Another problem lies, seemingly ironically, in the insufficient resources that can be expected to exist under any bloc grant program. Rather than yielding a situation in which providers must fiercely compete, the limited availability of resources means that coverage must be singular and spotty rather than multiple and potentially competitive. Thus, as Ruchlin (1977) has argued with regard to nursing homes, providers tend to have local monopolies in the service areas where they operate. Under these circumstances accountability generated by the market cannot be expected.

The Bloc Grant Option in Long-Term Care

The material in the beginning of this chapter is designed to serve as a basis for addressing the bloc grant option in long-term care. The issues raised, while generic in their presentation, will be of central importance should a bloc grant in long-term care be established, and many of them would surface in the political process that would precede adoption of that alternative. This section (1) presents an overall description of how such a bloc grant might be structured; (2) examines the likely effects implementation would have regarding such a grant program, such as (a) relative cost burdens, (b) distribution of services by client groups, (c) distribution of services by provider groups, (d) organizational issues particularly as they affect the DSA, and (e) political questions concerning the feasibility of a bloc grant's being enacted; and (3) concludes with a series of general recommendations as to what must be provided for and guarded against should the bloc grant alternative seriously be pursued.

Structure of a Bloc Grant in Long-Term Care

Within the general rubric "bloc grant," a number of variations are available in how a given program might be structured. The objectives of the law in question may vary in their specificity, a range of oversight authority may be given to federal officials, and the DSA may be presented with almost total latitude or be precluded from pursuing selected programmatic options. Additional variations come into play when consideration turns to a specific policy area such as long-term care. Different programmatic alternatives are possible in each of the central areas—clients, services, funding, administration, and enforcement. Basically, one combination of these different factors—believed to be a combination currently receiving greatest attention—is outlined and discussed here. Particular variations are entertained on occasion, but separate sets of alternatives are not discussed.

Provisions Related to Coverage. Long-term-care services supported through the bloc grant would be for persons who are disabled or over sixty-five years of age and suffering from chronic disabilities that impede their being able to function independently on a day-to-day basis. Eligibility would be liberalized from current long-term-care programs, but provisions would be included mandating eligibility for persons currently covered through Medicaid and Medicare. At their own choosing, the states would be permitted to fund long-term-care services for persons whose incomes are higher and whose disability (and discharge) status is less severe than persons currently covered.

States would also be free to cover a wide array of long-term-care-related services. The nonskilled-services restriction under Medicare long-term care would be liberalized or eliminated, and home-based services—perhaps with some restrictions—would not be made mandatory. As under present law, the states would be required to offer both skilled nursing and intermediate nursing care services to the eligible population. The mandating of some level of noninstitutional services would be the principal change in the overall services package from what it is at present.

Provisions Related to Funding. Funds under the proposed long-term-care program would be provided to the states on a formula basis. The formula would be based on the states' population and/or population that is over sixty-five and/or disabled and would also take into account some measure of programs now financing long-term-care services: Medicaid ($4.4 billion), Medicare ($440 million), Title XX ($66 million), and Title III of the Older Americans Act (perhaps $50 million). Transfers could also be made from relevant portions of housing, rehabilitation, and income programs, but they are not considered here.

Apart from the collapse of these separate authorities, the most important change the bloc grant would bring in the present funding system would be placing a cap on federal financial participation. This capping aspect represents a major change from the reimbursement mechanism under the Medicaid program—by far the largest public source of long-term-care funds. Presently under Medicaid, the states are reimbursed for a fixed percentage of the costs they incur, with the range from 50 percent to 83 percent for different states. This system is open-ended in that the federal government is obligated to pay this fixed percentage on whatever amount the states bill it for. Medicare's reimbursement is also open-ended and the mechanism bypasses the states altogether. Under the new system, the relatively modest long-term-care expenditures would be folded into the overall bloc grant, and also the capped Title XX currently funds (on a 75-25 matching basis) a wide array of social services for a broadly eligible population, and current expenditures related to long-term care would be transferred to the new program and to its formula allotment. Title III, also allocated on a formula basis, provides a variety of social services to the elderly through a network of substate agencies, and a bloc-grant alternative would necessitate placing some substantial portion of these funds under the aegis of the new designated agency.

A critical question in the funding of the new program would be at what dollar level would the federal cap be placed. Placing it at the present level of long-term-care funding under the existing programs would very quickly put an added burden on the states and other public treasuries and would mean additional out-of-pocket costs for those individuals who had anything in their pockets. Present demand for publicly supported long-term-care services is estimated by the CBO (1977) to be nearly three times the present supply (all of this for personal care, housing arrangements, home health and day care services). Future demand is expected to increase 40 percent between 1975 and 1985, and inflation cannot be expected to slow significantly, at least in the near term. All of these factors will serve to reduce significantly the proportion of the federal government's burden if the imposed cap is not somehow made "dynamic." A partial offset to the state burden will be present if the long-term bloc-grant program is established only after a national insurance program for acute care services is in place. This type of insurance program has the potential of freeing state resources that are now devoted to acute care under Medicaid. Whether those resources would or could be transferred to long-term care is extremely problematical.

Provisions Related to Administration. Conceptually, a bloc grant connotes a limited federal role in program administration and places the locus of program authority primarily with the states. How the states might choose to administer the program within their borders is very much their own choice. Federal law likely would require that certain sets of services be made available (statewide), that certain persons must be served, and that a single agency be designated to administer the program at the state level, but the ways in which the states might go from there is their own choice. Single-state agencies administering programs now folded into the bloc grant at the federal level, most likely would themselves be folded into the new DSA at the state level. But, conceivably they would remain outside and contract their services and those of their outside service constituencies with the DSA. The extent to which the new program would be meaningfully integrated at the state level would most likely be left as a state-level decision.

A number of options are possible concerning the substate administration and delivery of long-term-care services. The alternative involving the least change from present arrangements would have the DSA contracting with them reimbursing the variety of providers now in place and others that might develop. This localized and fragmented alternative would be much like the way in which state Title XX agencies currently administer the social services program. Other alternatives, potentially consistent with the bloc-grant framework, are the topics of other options papers being prepared: S/HMOs, community-based long-term-care organizations, and local case management or triage agencies. While none of these alternatives requires the presence of a state-level agency, they could operate in conjunction with such an agency whose role might be that of allocator, regulator, and oversight agent. Under any of these arrangements, the role of the state agency vis-à-vis substate agencies would be directly analogous to that of the relationship between federal and state agencies under the bloc grant alternatives outlined here. The state agency would ensure the provisions of certain services and establish procedural guidelines that the implementing agencies would be required to follow. State—and now substate—politics would be central in determining which of these mechanisms or combinations thereof would be established in the different states.

Anticipated Bloc Grant Effects

Establishment of a bloc grant to the states for long-term care would represent a major, though not revolutionary, change in the structuring of publicly financed long-term-care benefits. Without relatively precise estimates of what the federal government's financial share might be under the new arrangement and what guidelines may be established for the states, firm predictions about program consequences are impossible. Informed speculation can, however, be made, based on the earlier analysis and program outlines presented to this point.

Distribution of Costs. The stipulation that federal reimbursements to the states would be capped made in conjunction with the present long-term-care bloc grant option appears almost inevitably to translate into greater long-term-care costs being borne by the states. The likelihood that federal financing would maintain its relative place in the overall picture seems remote if the states cannot be reimbursed for a fixed percentage of their costs. No formula for federal funds lacking this feature will be written whereby growing demand can be offset in a manner equally beneficial to the states. Another option would be for the federal government to provide payments to the states per long-term-care recipient (controlling for levels of service, for instance), but that option has been ruled out for present purposes and, in any event, would probably be less advantageous to the states than the present Medicaid arrangement. Presumably, the formula devised would at least cover current federal contributions to state programs and add perhaps a bit more. But, unless it were upwardly revised on a continual and frequent basis (as Title XX has not been), state costs would increase on a relative as well as an absolute basis.

As already indicated, an assumption is being made for present purposes that a national health insurance program would be in effect at the time a long-term-care bloc grant program would be instituted. This insurance program would presumably relieve the states of a very large portion of their Medicaid expenditures devoted to purposes other than long-term care—approximately 60 percent of the total on a national basis. Under these circumstances, the federal government may well expect the states to devote some portion of this considerable relief for long-term-care purposes. As the federal government cannot direct states how to spend their revenues, it would have to make spending stipulations part of the requirements that the states must meet in receiving federal assistance through the bloc grant. For this to work, the amount of federal dollars would have to be relatively substantial in order that some states do not choose simply to opt out of the program (as Arizona continues to do with Medicaid).

The potential problem of adequate state participation will be aggravated by growing restiveness among taxpayers in various states. One can picture the announcement that the federal government is taking over all public health care costs (except long-term care) and taxpayers' being told that the largest single item in (many) state budgets has magically disappeared. To then be told that nearly half of that amount cannot be saved because of the seemingly innocuous entry "long-term care" will not sit well. Among the possible consequences are that the federal share will have to be greater than anticipated, that adequate state funds will not be made available and services will be cut, or that the states will agree that a half a loaf is better than none. While the combination of national health insurance and largely state-financed long-term-care programs appears on its face to be a very good deal for the states, it may not appear as such to taxpayers who may simply not believe that care for the old and disabled could possibly cost so much, or perhaps, be worth it.

Given the assumption that some form of national health insurance will be in place and given concerns about spending and taxes at the state level, a great probability exists that the states would try to push long-term-care clients into the national system whenever possible. The states would save money and providers would receive higher reimbursements because the patients would, by definition, be seen as receiving expensive acute care services. In addition to this move's placing a further drain on the federal program, it would also reinforce the institutional bias in long-term care. For this ploy to work, clients would have to be receiving the skilled and intensive services offered only in hospitals or skilled nursing facilities. Were the latter type of institution not eligible for reimbursement through the national health insurance program, pressures on placing long-term-care clients in hospitals would still remain, however inappropriate that type of care might be.

Folding into the new system Title XX and Title III long-term-care funds will be of no particular interest to most state officials or taxpayers, but it is likely to appease affected officials and constituencies. The volume of funds in these programs is small compared to Medicaid, but these programs have funded most of the noninstitutional services that currently exist. The reasons for expected resistance are dealt with to a greater length in a subsequent section, but here it can be simply noted that keeping these programs separate from the overall bloc grant—however wise that might be for some purposes—would result in funds under the bloc grant being spent almost entirely for institutional services. The cost pressures will probably be severe enough that adoption of significant noninstitutional services in a program domain where they have been foreign and ancillary is unlikely.

Depending on the magnitude of federal funding, the monetary and "in-kind" costs borne by older and disabled persons and their relatives will increase. The effect of federal/state funding's not keeping base with the essential demand must hit these individuals and could be very substantial given that Medicaid pays upward of 90 percent of nursing home costs in some states. Lessening availability of public funds raises economic and ethical issues concerning family responsibility and quality of care and life-threatening issues for persons with severe chronic conditions. That families—for a variety of well-known reasons—will become less able (and perhaps willing) to continue their assistance may put added pressures on public programs at a time when state concerns and federal funds are being directed into other areas. Finally, a reduced federal-funding role will offer no relief for the heavy out-of-pocket expenses the chronically ill and disabled must pay on their own. Present estimates indicate that half of long-term-care expenses are borne privately, with nearly 90 percent being out of pocket. The bloc-grant alternative and the politics that may surround its implementation offer no relief to this heavy burden and its rather draconian "spend-down" consequences.

If the assumption that the federal cap on long-term-care funds to the states will fall behind legitimate demand is correct, the financial consequences for all other factors affected by long-term-care policy are not favorable. Reduced federal funding's also being accompanied by a bloc-grant structure creates further problems. States would have increased responsibility for program direction, and high on their agenda would be devising ways of how to avoid having the bulk of the added fiscal burden placed on them. The federal government's picking up acute care costs now borne by the states opens the possibility for increased state effort in long-term care, but it certainly does not guarantee it. The states may in fact call fiscal relief in long-term care "national health insurance."

Organizational Issues. The enactment of a long-term-care bloc grant—involving a cap on federal financing and folding in now free-standing federal categorical-grant programs—will have major repercussions in the state capitols. One need only picture the meeting at which the governor announces to a series of single-state agencies that their functions have been eliminated or drastically curtailed and that some but not all of them will be joining another agency that currently does not exist or that exists but is unliked. In the presence of certain conditions to be mentioned momentarily, the long-run effect might be salutory; however, the near-term disruptions as affected parties resist or adapt will be chaotic. Consumers as well as bureaucrats and providers could easily be adversely affected.

As discussed generically and at some length in Part I, the most critical organizational element will be the formal authority and informal support that finally rests with the designated long-term-care agency. An agency that finds itself with limited authority through legislation and an indifferent or hostile state administration in the face of resentment from dispossessed state agencies and demands of providers for contractual safeguards is going to be very hardpressed. If each of these extremes emerges, the agency will be unable to act and the program will be a disaster.

All of this chaos need not come to pass. The federal legislation must and probably will contain provisions mandating certain basic services and coverage for the very poor and the most vulnerable. In such matters the law will also require considerable state financing. (It is assumed the federal share will remain sufficiently large to induce the states into meeting this set of minimum requirements.) At the same time it must be noted that to the extent the federal government imposes requirements, the grant becomes less bloc and more categorical. Restrictions along the lines suggested here, if multiplied, would make this option look increasingly like an expanded Medicaid program with contained federal funding. If the concept "bloc grant" is to be taken at all literally, limits will be put on specific federal program requirements with all of the potential dangers in such limitations.

Variability among states makes specifying how the new agency may be viewed and supported difficult. The imperatives of elected office and the nonpervasive concerns with governent spending hold out little prospect for expecting support for expanded and liberalized state long-term-care programs. At the same time, even the new wave of neoconservative politicians claim that social welfare benefits for those "who really need them" will not be curtailed. They go on to say that it is fraud and inefficiencies they will root out that, if it were confined to that, would be welcome in long-term care. It seems unlikely, however, that any elected officials will be found favoring major new funding commitments in any social welfare programs in the absence of a very favorable federal reimbursement policy. Within social welfare, long-term care is an unlikely area for governors and legislators to single out for demonstrating their ongoing concern for the disadvantaged. And the incentive to move in this direction by virtue of liberal federal financing appears precluded by the federal cap assumed to be placed on long-term-care funding. What appears more likely, as discussed previously, is that state leadership will encourage program administrators to define chronic conditions as acute problems, thereby being able to place long-term-care patients under the national health insurance program.

Demands from providers on the DSA will be inconsistent with the pressures coming from above. Nursing homes and other institutions that may be categorically excluded from national health insurance participation will demand rate relief and continue to argue for the construction of new facilities. Demands by workers in these facilities for higher wages and improved working conditions will continue to grow. In each of these cases, the threat to refuse to take new patients or to strike will be present if relief is not forthcoming. Providers or would-be providers of noninstitutional services—backed by some consumers and professionals—will at the same time be calling for the development and explosion of these options. Using the argument that such services are needed, desired, appropriate, and potentially cost-efficient, these people will press for these services and those who provide them to be eligible for third-party payments on a parity basis with providers of institutional care.

The position of the DSA will be, at minimum, trying to mediate among the contending forces and, one must hope, to provide some leadership and direction as the states become more directly responsible for the administration of long-term-care services. Their ability to lead in this charged environment will be a function of their internal resources (executive direction, skilled personnel, substantive knowledge, political acumen) and outside support from some mix of the claimants. Provider groups and others who have been the principal Medicaid constituency will be best positioned to influence the agency and will, in turn, offer it their support if their prerogatives are maintained. Other groups will offer support if some commitment—and shortly thereafter, tangible evidence—exists that the DSA will assist in their development and utilize their services. Limited commitments may generate support that, in turn, will provide a platform for further positive actions.

The organizational problem will be for the DSA to develop some level of autonomy and cohesion so that it does not find itself endlessly buffeted by contending outside forces and a disenchanted internal staff. The latter may be a considerable problem where states do choose to consolidate agencies as well as programs. Meeting the concerns of the previously separate agency personnel who had identified with the elderly and disabled groups while maintaining other sources of support in the presence of only limited resources will be a difficult task.

Some of the presumed advantages of the bloc grant concept may be hard to carry out in practice under these conditions. Heretofore, separate programs will be brought together under a long-term-care bloc grant, but their being effectively consolidated and integrated is another question. Personnel identifying with particular program components will be wary of integration attempts, and this wariness will be particularly true of the smaller and newer places fearful of being swallowed up. What may result in the absence of strong agency leadership will be an uncomfortable confederation of long-term-care actors, each concerned with its relative standing vis-a-vis the others. These concerns may preclude a related advantage associated with bloc grants, that of program flexibility. Given that the new program is imposed on programmatic territory that is already occupied, very little movement and change may be necessary. This movement could take either the form of border skirmishes or could result in a "domain-consensus" pattern in which all parties tacitly agree not to interfere with each other's operations.

These pressures and concerns apparently may also negate the (political) institution building associated with the bloc grant concept. Central to that notion is an agency's being so positioned and supported that it develops bureaucratic, political, and financial resources sufficient to provide it with the autonomy and cohesion necessary to direct the policy-implementation process. As the scenario plays out in long-term care, the DSA may find such development beyond its grasp. The near-term problem will be to keep the agency from being coopted or disrupted by the contending public and private interests seeking to push it and long-term-care policy in different directions.

Finally, the presumed virtue of a more open decision-making process associated with bloc grants seems unlikely to play out according to form. There are few areas where the chances for meaningful consumer participation are less likely to be effective than in long-term care. Physical and mental impairments and longstanding social isolation create almost overwhelming obstacles to many of the old and some of the younger disabled consumers of long-term-care services. At the level of providers, the competition and compromise that might yield responsive policies will suffer from the particularistic concerns, uneven access and resources, and limited pool of funds. Entrenched interests in the long-term-care field—most notably nursing homes—will dominate the participatory process, with the newly developing community-based groups struggling to maintain their place. These latter groups will already have seen the enactment of the bloc grant and the creation of the DSA as steps that bode ill for them. While it may not usually be thought of in these terms, placing the locus of authority of a single agency in the narrower jurisdictional boundaries of the states will make domination by a single interest such as nursing homes easier to come by. Long-term-care decisions left to a nominally open process at the state level will not yield the kinds of changes around which considerable professional consensus has been reached in recent years.

Effect on Providers. Much that can be said here follows directly from the last set of observations. Development of a bloc-grant system, in the absence of a strong DSA, will serve to maintain the present institutional bias in long-term care. Institutional providers are the largest in number, most highly organized, and will have greater access to public officials both in the DSA and above it than other provider groups in long-term care. In the absence of the language mandating the provision of noninstitutional services and specifying what portion of resources must be devoted to such services, the present system is unlikely to change significantly in most states.

Providers and advocates of other types of services will try to maintain the impetus toward integrated community-based services but are likely to find little protection in bloc grant legislation. In states such as New York where these services are relatively well developed, one may expect that current levels can be roughly maintained, but in that large number of states where noninstitutional services are barely off the ground, service development will be difficult. The principal cause for optimism in these areas—particularly predominantly rural areas—will lie in the scarcity of all kinds of long-term-care services including institutional ones. Under these circumstances, competition may be more balanced. Also more likely in these settings is that constituency-based public agencies—particularly the state and area agencies on aging—may be in a relatively advantageous position as contrasted with their standing in more urbanized areas of the country.

While these essentially political factors suggest that significant growth in noninstitutional services will be difficult to come by under the bloc grant arrangement, it is important to note that, formally at least, the bloc grant does remove federal requirements that helped spawn the growth of a long-term-care system heavily biased toward institutional care. The necessity for obtaining waivers on a piecemeal basis, such as in the Triage, Monroe County, and Wisconsin Community Care cases, will no longer be necessary. The bloc-grant alternative is, at best, only a halfway step toward seeing the system move away from its institutional orientation. Clearly, more direct and purposive legislation could be devised for ensuring the development of community-based, noninstitutional alternatives. Political and cost considerations suggest that enactment of legislation mandating and funding specific community-based options will be very difficult to bring about, but on program grounds that does not make the bloc grant alternative any more attractive.

A final and more optimistic observation is the political and programmatic weight that should be given to noninstitutional service because of its known and presumed advantages as a service delivery mechanism. That case can be quite effectively argued now, and one would expect that further research as to consumer satisfaction and functioning will add to the body of evidence that speaks for such services. Should research also be able to isolate conditions under which noninstitutional services are cost-effective as well as socially desirable, the case can be made more strongly yet. By itself, such knowledge will not overcome all of the political difficulties found with the bloc-grant alternative, but reliable information about services effectiveness can be of considerable use even in a highly politicized environment.

Effect on Consumers. In the short run, one would not expect implementation of the bloc grant alternative to bring about major changes in long-term care at the point of delivery. Initially, the major change will take place farther up the administrative chain. Beyond that, at least two sets of pressures will be at work that could have very different effects on the consumer population. On the one hand, the pressures and concerns would make the long-term-care system more akin to welfare than is even now the case. Cost-conscious state officials will probably try to impose strict income and disability criteria that consumers would have to meet in order to be eligible for state-supported services. While these officials would not disagree that many of the old and disabled persons have legitimate need for long-term-care services, liberalizing eligibility criteria would generate demand that could not be met within the budgetary constraints that officials face and/or create. On the other hand, to liberalize eligibilty criteria and then provide insufficient funds, does not expand services and, in fact, creates equity problems of its own.

This type of move leads to the second set of pressures. Many providers will seek out consumers who are able to pay for some or all of their own care and/or have relatively minor disabilities. Service costs are lower, and reimbursement may be the same as for persons who are more severely disabled. Under a state bloc-grant system, providers can be expected to seek out persons who are better off being eligible for state-supported services; the providers could then target their recruitment and service areas toward these individuals. The question, of course, is what then becomes of the poor and severely disabled persons when services are going to this other group? Presumably, providers and the state as well would try to place them in facilities covered through the national health insurance system. The system could not go totally in this direction, but the pressures would be there, and the legislation as interpreted at the state level might not adequately guard against a considerable amount of this creaming from taking place. The larger issue here is where on a continuum from welfare to entitlement the emphasis of the long-term-care bloc grant will be placed. The stigma and other effects of means-tested programs are clearly undesirable, but they do serve to target resources on those who, at least on income grounds, are the most in need. An entitlement program allows disabled persons access to public services independent of income, but where such a program is underfunded—as it will be under the federally capped bloc-grant alternative—persons who are worst off may get left out. That presently large numbers of persons are in need of services and are not receiving them suggests further that liberalization of eligibility criteria in the absence of major new resources would lead toward "negative redistribution" of long-term-care benefits. The fundamental problem is, of course, money, but as long as it remains insufficient, safeguards for those most in need must be maintained. In most states such restrictions likely would be kept even if provisions under the bloc grant did not require it, but the possibility of inappropriate allocation remains.

Political Feasibility. Possibly many of the arguments made here about the merits of a bloc grant in long-term care will remain irrelevant and untested because of the political uncertainty that awaits a true bloc grant proposal. Considerable opposition will spring up in the face of such a proposal, but the long-term-care grant's being linked to federal assumption of acute care costs may be sufficient to overcome the opposition.

In the case of other bloc grant programs, the major source of political support has come from governors, mayors, and their offices. Bloc grants give these officials a greater say in how federal monies are spent, more control over line officials at the state and local levels, and a better opportunity to establish projects in settings where the political pay-off is relatively high.

Long-term-care policy, as it is presently constituted, limits many of the political advantages a bloc grant could bring. Long-term-care consumers have little political currency, new provider groups cannot be indulged without alienating other groups, and the designated agency will likely be a place of contending factions rather than a locus of program control. More generally, long-term care is a prototypical area in which governors would like to pass responsibility up the federal ladder rather than finding it placed in their laps. What they in turn would do under these circumstances is lay off all the problems on the DSAs, thereby creating many of the program problems discussed earlier. What, of course, makes the option being considered here especially unpalatable is the expected cap on federal funding. To be given more direct responsibility for a politically unrewarding policy area with the added likelihood of more limited federal funding is a combination no governor could reasonably be expected to want.

The only way state leadership could be expected to accept the bloc grant notion would be to make clearly a part of the package deal the federal government's picking up other existing state health care costs. That idea is being envisaged here, and on the right terms it might be acceptable to the states. The federal government's picking up all nonlong-term-care Medicaid costs would more than compensate in the near term for the added burden brought on by the federal cap on long-term-care spending. Under these circumstances the states might accept a maintenance- (and expansion) of-effort clause that would have to be part of the bloc grant. The scenario's unfolding like this would be very reminiscent of the process leading to Title XX: the states accepted a cap on federal funding when it was attached to the general-revenue-sharing bill, which gave them considerably greater relief (Mott 1976).

Long-term care is an area in which the bloc grant option would get decidedly mixed reviews from affected private interests. Institutional providers might favor it on the grounds that they would be able to exercise disproportionate influence on how the states allocated long-term-care funds, and nascent providers of alternative types of care could be expected to oppose the plan on the same grounds. Professionals and others might also favor the bloc grant idea on the grounds that it would eliminate federal requirements that have directed most funds toward institutions, but the contention here is that their believing a relatively unrestricted bloc grant to the states would necessarily change that situation is misguided.

Considerable opposition would come from categorical-grant-program interests, which would be administratively folded into the bloc grant program. They would lose the separate recognition and protection they now enjoy through their own federal programs and could only expect to occupy a relatively minor place under the DSA. Individual and organized constituents of these agencies would also voice opposition for the same reasons. The argument in both of these cases is that innovative and needed programs would suffer irreparable damage if housed with the major institutional programs.

These arguments would surface at the federal as well as the state level. The Older Americans Act has developed a large number of congressional advocates who get a great deal more mileage from standing for the dignity of senior citizens than they would from a functional program targeted on the vulnerable and impaired elderly. The political problems in the case of Title XX would be a bit different. Title XX came into being as the result of a fragile coalition of governors (seeking relatively unencumbered social services funding) and social service organizations (seeking guarantees that the funds would be spent only for purposes associated with social welfare). At least the second part of that coalition would react strongly against any foray aimed at categorizing part of those funds for a function such as long-term care. Were this reaction to occur, others would immediately demand the same kind of earmarking of funds for their program areas; rather than confront this unravelling and its consequences, the coalition can be expected to strongly oppose the initial encroachment.

As with many aspects of the bloc grant alternative, a precise estimate of chances for enactment cannot be made in the absence of more precise information about what the final form of the grant might be. On balance, it appears that the most affected interests would oppose it, but the grant's being tied to a proposal in which the federal goverment picks up acute care costs might overwhelm opposition from these sources. Under these conditions, long-term care would become only one place of a much larger undertaking.

Conclusion

Should a bloc grant program in long-term care be proposed and implemented, the following issues will remain critical:

Means for ensuring that persons currently being served cannot be dropped from the system;

Service options now largely confined to programs' being folded into the bloc-grant system not be pressured out of existence;

Mechanisms in place that assure acceptable quality-of-care levels;

A range of service alternatives available so that consumers and/or case managers have reasonable choice;

Safeguards in place so that consumers are not forced into inappropriate settings financed by the federal government;

Most basic of all, that the federal government has some meaningful way of enforcing the legislative and regulatory provisions contained in federal legislation.

Notes

1. On these and other issues related to federalism and grants-in-aid, see Deil S. Wright, *Understanding Intergovernmental Relations* (North Scituate, Mass.: Duxbury Press, 1978); and Michael D. Reagan, *The New Federalism* (New York: Oxford University Press, 1972).

2. T. Sanford. 1968. *Storm Over the States* (Chicago: Rand McNally), p. 50.

3. An excellent discussion of the knowledge problem as it relates to choice making in the soical services is found in Melvin Mogulof, *Making Social Service Choices at the State Level: Practice and Problems in Four States* (Washington, D.C.: Urban Institute, 1973).

4. An analysis of this problem in the social services is found in Robert B. Hudson, "Mixed Implementation Models and Title XX," *Urban and Social Change Review* 13 (Winter 1980):6-13.

5. For an excellent discussion of the meaning and import of this distinction, see James W. Fesler, "Approaches to the Understanding of Decentralization," *Journal of Politics* 27 (August 1965):536-566.

References

Eisenstadt, S.N. 1959. "Bureaucracy, Bureaucratization, and Debureaucratization." *Administrative Science Quarterly* 1 (December):302-320.

Mayhew, D. 1974. *Congress: The Electoral Connection*. New Haven: Yale University Press.

Mott, P. 1976. *Meeting Human Needs: The Social and Political History of Title XX*. Columbus, Ohio: National Conference on Social Welfare.

Ruchlin, H. 1977. "A New Strategy for Regulating Long-Term Care Facilities." *Journal of Health Politics, Policy and Law* 2 (Summer):190-211.

Schattschnieder, E.E. 1960. *The Semi-Sovereign People*. New York: Holt, Rinehart and Winston.

Seidman, H. 1975. *Politics, Position, and Power*. New York: Oxford University Press.

U.S. Congressional Budget Office. 1977. *Long-Term Care for the Elderly and Disabled*. Washington, D.C.: Government Printing Office, p. ix.

4 A Compulsory National Long-Term-Care-Insurance Program

Christine E. Bishop

At the root of current concern with our nation's policy toward long-term care is dissatisfaction with the amount and distribution of resources supplied through private markets and public programs to disabled and chronically ill individuals. The current distribution of resources does much to determine what daily life is like over the years for a person with functional impairment and/or chronic ill health. Our dissatisfaction with current allocation can be seen philosophically in two distinct perspectives.

The first perspective is somewhat altruistic. Many people in our society are shocked and dismayed by the hardships current policy forces on some individuals: the residents of low-quality nursing homes, the elderly struggling to live independently despite handicaps and poverty, the overburdened families caring for disabled members to avoid their placement in institutions. A look at the distribution of resources and the accompanying variation in well-being across individuals who differ by disability, income, location, family situation, and personal preferences indicates that better distribution might be possible. Clearly, the situation in which the disabled find themselves depends on a number of personal characteristics:

Income level: If their income level is high, they are able to pay for desired care themselves; if it is low, they are eligible for Medicaid assistance. People of intermediate wealth and income may spend all their assets in purchasing care or go without care.

Location: Public support for disability-related services varies across states, and geographic areas vary in their supply of services. For example, some areas have been aggressive in securing funds for elderly housing, some states have long waiting lists for nursing home placement, some Title XX programs actively provide home care, and states have varying eligibility criteria for Medicaid.

Nature of disability: End-stage renal disease immediately qualifies a disabled person for Medicare; people with chronic or terminal conditions with little promise of rehabilitation have difficulty obtaining long-term-care services under Medicare; people whose condition does not require hospitalization are not eligible for Medicare nursing home and home health services; people with personal care needs, in contrast to those with nursing or medical needs, are eligible only for lower cost institutions and less generous home services, although meeting their needs may be as expensive as meeting the nursing needs of others.

Family situation: The private resources available for care of the disabled are likely to be greater if they have living relatives. These resources include the time of unpaid family members, as well as family funds. The willingness of public programs to assume the care of a disabled person is lower if he or she has family with monetary resources.

Personal preferences: Individuals with the same disability status, income, and family situation may prefer different living arrangements. Currently, public programs pay for room and board as well as medical and personal care for disabled poor elderly who choose nursing home care and provide only occasional home visits for those choosing to live at home.

Implicit in any public choice of a long-term-care strategy is a determination of whose situation should be improved, how much benefit will be provided, and how much the public is willing to pay to change benefit distribution in this way.

The second perspective on long-term-care policy is in a sense more selfish: any one of us faces a probability of becoming disabled, of becoming impoverished by the cost of our own care, and of finding ourselves without family support or adequate living arrangements. At present an individual has little means to insure against these eventualities, and current policies toward the disabled are unlikely to make us sanguine about our own fate should we become disabled. Many people as individuals would probably be willing to pay individually to make their own future well-being more certain, and for many people this may be a more compelling reason for support of long-term-care expenditures than assuring the well-being of others.

It is argued in this chapter that a compulsory national long-term-care-insurance program has the potential to shift the distribution of resources better to meet social goals of improved quality of life for disabled people and that such a program can provide individual protection against certain risks that the private-insurance market fails to offer. The chapter argues for long-term-care insurance based on the desirability and unavailability of individual private coverage. Thus, support for publicly provided insurance against long-term care expenditures need not rest on altruism alone.

The first section of the chapter, "Long-Term-Care-Benefit Provision As Insurance," places disability benefits in an insurance framework and specifies those events against which consumers wish to insure. While the risk of disability itself is the main event determining disability-related expense, insurance protection would be less costly if insured expenditures were also seen as determined by the uncertain availability of family personal care and community social support. The next section, "Failure of the Private Market for Long-Term-Care Insurance," explores the reasons that insurance for disability benefit has not been offered by private-insurance companies. The section that follows, "Design Issues for a Public Long-Term-Care-Insurance Program," presents several issues that must be resolved in the design of a public long-term-care-benefit insurance program. The discussion focuses on methods to determine how much service will be reimbursed for disabled beneficiaries. Three alternatives are contrasted: (1) payment for all covered services up to specified limits, (2) payment only for the amount and type of service prescribed by needs assessment, and (3) payment for services chosen by consumers. The last section specifies "A Prototype Copayment Long-Term-Care-Insurance Plan" and concludes with "Predicting Impacts of a National Long-Term-Care-Insurance Program," a framework for evaluating this prototype and other alternative long-term-care-policy changes.

Long-Term-Care-Benefit Provision as Insurance

Economists have argued persuasively that an individual's well-being over a lifetime is enhanced if he or she is able to buy actuarily fair insurance against risks of expense, when spending would be desired only in specific probabilistic situations (Arrow 1963; Zeckhauser 1973). When there is a small chance of a large loss of well-being, which could be compensated for by a money (or service) benefit paid only if the unpleasant event occurs, a rational consumer should prefer to lose a small amount for sure (an insurance premium) in exchange for the insurer's promise to pay if the event happens, rather than keeping the insurance premium and facing the risk of a large loss. What is sold by the insurer and bought by the insured is called a *contingent claim*. The claim states, "If event A occurs, the company will pay $x."[1] In this framework, it is necessary to specify the contingencies or events that consumers wish to insure against; and the occurrence of the insured-for event must be clearly discernible to observers, so that it is clear when a payoff is due under the contract. The payoff must also be specified in advance.

Protection from the heavy expense of disability-related services fits this classic insurance framework. Every individual faces a significant probability of becoming disabled at some time in his or her life. While no insurance policy can guarantee the replacement of a lost limb, eye, or functional capacity, a monetary payoff can compensate, at least in part, for direct money losses due to disability. Two types of losses should be distinguished here: loss of income due to inability to work, and losses due to the expense of overcoming or ameliorating the disabling condition.[2] The insurance considered here is of the second type only; it would replace money spent on disability-related services. Separating these two types of insurance is reasonable, first because insurance replacing the earned income of disabled individuals is widely available in the private insurance market, and second because the population of major concern for long-term-care needs and services is the elderly, who rely mainly on unearned income. The probability of needing disability-related services at some time in one's lifetime is not small. For example, estimates indicate that one in four people over sixty-five will make use of a particularly expensive service—nursing home care—at some time in their lives (Kastenbaum and Candy 1973; Palmore 1976). Nevertheless, this probability is far from 100 percent, and the timing of the need for expenditure is very uncertain. Moreover, the amount a disabled person would wish to spend to compensate for a disability is variable and may be very large (CBO 1977). This means that individuals cannot effectively prepare to pay disability expenses: the timing and amount of the expenses are unknown, and one may not need to incur them at all. Thus the problem of disability-related long-term-care expense is appropriate for treatment as insurance and is not simply a reflection of inadequate income levels of elderly people.

Protection from unpredictable disability-related expense entails that long-term-care services should be paid for while a person is disabled. The amount a disabled person would wish to spend to compensate for the disability depends not only on the nature and extent of the disability but also on the price of services at the time the disability occurs, the ability of family members to provide personal care and social support services, and the ability of the living situation to support the independent function of a disabled individual. All of these aspects are subject to uncertainty. It is assumed here that the risks due to inflation will be borne by the insurer, parallel to acute health care insurance where needed services are paid for under insurance plans. The risks of disability and of disability with loss of family and community support will be dealt with by delineating two possible insurance approaches. The first is a straightforward approach in which a specific service benefit is provided when a specific disability is present. The second is a more complex approach in which services provided are contingent both on disability and on other factors, specifically presence of family and appropriateness of living situation, which would affect the value to the individual of service benefits given disability. It will be argued that the second type of insurance policy, while more complex to administer, will be more efficient in distributing well-being across various future uncertain states.

Benefits Contingent on Disability Alone

In the most general sense, the key uncertain events to be insured for are expenditures determined by the beneficiary's particular disabling condition and by the duration of disability. Expense needed for a disabled person to realize his or her potential for independent function is different depending on the nature of the disabilities (inability to walk, inability to perform simple manual tasks, incontinence, difficulty in communicating, and so on), and also depends on the length of time the disabling conditions hold. Thus, one form of disability insurance might specify a set of services to be paid for per month given Condition A, another set for Condition B, and so on; or, rather than specifying actual services, the amount of payment could be left up to a technical team, who would examine the patient and certify the claim for benefits. This approach applies the acute health insurance model to long-term-care benefits, including home nursing, congregate housing, nursing home care, and the like. If the client is certified to be in need of service, based on the presence of disability alone, the claim would be paid by the insurance company.

Benefits Contingent on Joint Risks of
Disability and Other Events

If individuals could buy their own disability services insurance, they might seek cheaper insurance packages better tailored to their own expected use of disability services. The amount of expense one would expect to incur to compensate for a given disabling condition depends on other uncertain factors besides the condition itself and its duration.

A hypothetical insurance policy can be designed to insure against three types of risks:

1. The risk of incurring major treatment and personal care expense because of disability, this expense is contingent on the extent and duration of disability;
2. The risk of being disabled without family, which increases one's desire to purchase personal care services;
3. The risk that community and living arrangements will be rendered unsuitable by a disabling condition, increasing one's demand for social support services.

The contrast to be drawn is that an insurance program whose benefit is based on the presence of a disabling condition *alone* must provide the same service benefit to disabled people living in close-knit communities and handicapped-accessible housing as to people living in physical and social isolation. The purchaser of insurance will be better off with a policy whose benefit package is contingent on these risky future states of the world as well as on disability so that, for example, he will receive a smaller personal care benefit if he is lucky enough to have family who can assist him when disabled, and a greater service benefit if he is without family. In contrast to an insurance policy providing services according to the disabling condition and ignoring the ability of family and living situation to meet disability needs, limitations on benefits that take family care into account will save the buyer premium dollars. Under such a limited plan, the individual in effect agrees in advance to accept benefits contingent not only on disability but also on family and living situation. Benefits can usefully be divided into three categories of service: treatment, personal care, and social support, which includes aspects of room and board services.

Treatment Benefit. Treatment expense can be predicted most directly by looking forward to the amount of service one would want to consume given specific disabling conditions: if Condition A, then 2.1 hours of nursing care per week would be desired; if Condition B, three physical therapy sessions per week, and so on. We could assume that the rational insurance buyer and seller would be willing to specify service for each possible condition in an insurance contract. An alternative is to follow the path of acute health insurance and stipulate that treatment prescribed by a specified professional "gatekeeper" would be paid for. This portion of the insurance package is not contingent on family situation.

Personal Care Benefit. Personal care expense that a private individual would want to insure for depends on two uncertainties: disabling condition and family situation. The buyer of private insurance would be aware that if he insured for maximum personal care spending, based on disabling condition, his premium would be higher than if he made the insurance company's obligation contingent on both his condition and his family situation at the time of disability. Theoretically, it could be specified in the policy that the ability of his spouse and other household members to provide personal care would be assessed at the time he became disabled and that the insurance company would be liable for the difference between this amount and need, as computed based on his condition. Such a "personal care deductible," with the first so many hours of care to be provided by family members if they are available, allows direct insurance against the possibility that one would be left without family to meet personal care needs.

Social Support Benefit. In like manner, payment for needed assistance with household management, cleaning, chores, transportation, letter writing, and so on could be made contingent not only on disability-determined need, but on the ability of family and community to provide assistance. In this case, family and living situation (near a bus line? in an apartment with other people? near reasonable restaurants? involved in community activities?) could be taken into account along with disability. In theory, the individual would see himself as insuring against changes in his community that would reduce his ability to function if disabled.

Benefits Involving Room-and-Board Expense. A difficult question for disability insurance is the coverage of living expenses that people incur whether disabled or not. Having lived all his life in a fifth-floor walk-up or a suburban house with two acres of lawn and an icy front walk, how can our rational insurance buyer insure against the possibility that disability will strike, making a change of location or architectural alterations desirable if he is to maintain his potential for independence? In a world with no inflation, the rational purchaser of insurance has presumably already arranged to meet expected "standard" needs for income through a combination of disability income insurance, social security, employer pensions, and savings. Disability insurance payments for altered housing, meals-on-wheels, elderly housing, room and board in a congregate living arrangement, or room and board in a nursing home should ideally be for the difference between what the individual expected to spend anyway and the housing and/or meals required by his disability. If the purchaser insures for the whole cost, for example, of housing for the elderly, the insurance company would pay all his housing expenses if he becomes disabled, and he would be able to spend his former rent check on other things. The expected value of this extra consumption if disabled is unlikely to be worth the extra premium cost of full room and board coverage to an individual insuring privately against pure disability expenses.

Comparison of Insurance Approaches

Contrasting the two types of insurance plans presented here is useful: the simple disability expenditure insurance and the more complex expenditure insurance which makes the payoff contingent on family and living situation as well as disability. Both types follow basic tenets of insurance in that rules could be laid out for determining when the insured-for events have occurred and what the payoff should be. The first alternative, in which the risk insured against is disability-related need for services, is more straightforward because family and community situation need not be considered. Under such a policy, if disability of a certain type occurs, the insurance company pays for prescribed home health visits; if another type occurs, then the company pays the full cost of prescribed nursing home care; if a third type of disability occurs, then congregate housing is paid for by the insurer. Clearly, such a simplified policy would be much more expensive than the second alternative, a policy insuring jointly against loss of family support and unsuitability of living situation, along with the disability. The simple disability policy does not allow the married individual with children to economize on premiums by promising that family members will provide some care, if available, and also makes the disabled person eligible for a full living-arrangement change, no matter what the living situation was at the onset of the disability.

Failure of the Private Market for Long-Term-Care Insurance

Insurance policies covering expenditures on long-term-care services for chronic conditions are not widely available in the private insurance market. Some private health insurance plans do cover some medically related long-term-care services that substitute for acute services like extended-care-facility care and home health visits, but these plans are strictly limited in duration. Private acute health expenditure insurance does not cover personal care and social support services, which may be necessary for maximization of independent function of the disabled, and most important, private coverage for disability-related services is not widely available to retired people, who are the heaviest users of long-term care (Feder and Holahan 1979).

Foresighted people have the opportunity to purchase insurance to protect themselves from many types of possible future losses. Thus, it may seem puzzling that the insurance industry, able to supply life, home, automobile, acute health, and disability income-replacement insurance, has not offered insurance against future disability-related expenditures. A number of reasons may be advanced for the unavailability of this type of insurance. First, the discrepancy between the income of potential purchasers and their actuarially fair premium over the life cycle could curtail demand for short-term coverage, although this need not be a problem under lifetime-coverage plans. Second, uncertainty about future prices for care would add substantially to the insurer's risk under a lifetime-coverage plan and may be an insurmountable problem for private coverage. Third, administration of a lifetime-coverage package would be costly without widespread coverage of the population. Fourth, the floor under long-term-care services provided by current public programs reduces private demand for disability coverage. And finally, two classic problems of insurance—adverse selection and moral hazard—may be greater for insurance against chronic conditions than for other types of insurance.

Synchronization of Premium, Expected
Payout, and Income

The timing of the expected value of disability-related expense and income may reduce demand for insurance sold on a year-to-year basis. People face an increasing probability of becoming disabled as they age, meaning that an actuarially fair premium for disabling conditions must rise with age, which is when income typically falls. If life span could be predicted, the rational individual could budget future disability insurance premiums by saving for this expense during working years. However, people also face an increasing probability of death as they age. The individual who is prepared to pay the full disability insurance premium through, say, age 100 will probably have saved too much. In a sense, the individual should purchase an annuity that covers his expected future premiums, thus taking into account his probability of dying. This would be equivalent to lifetime coverage, purchased either through a one-time payment or, as in whole-life insurance, a level premium, designed to be much too high in early years and much less than actuarial value in later years. Under such a private plan, someone buying disability benefit insurance at age 35 would contract for a lower per-year price for lifetime coverage than would a new 65-year-old purchaser. Thus it seems that the timing issue in itself should not be an insurmountable obstacle to an industry that provides lifetime-coverage life insurance.

Inflation

A lifetime service benefit policy would insure individuals against the vagaries of future inflation, guaranteeing their ability to purchase needed services in the future, no matter what their real income or the price of services. While attractive to the buyer, such insurance represents more risk than insurance companies are currently willing to take on; insurance policies with potentially distant payoffs (for example, life insurance) have payoffs denominated in money, not real, terms. In addition, a policy that promises to pay for the difference between the living situation at the time of disablement and the living arrangement appropriate to disability would involve even more uncertainty, since it would, in essence, be insuring a part of real future income if disabled. For example, the insurance company would promise to pay the increment of congregate housing rent over an individual's actual housing expense when he became disabled. Since a specific monetary amount budgeted for housing might pay for a luxury retirement condominium at age sixty-five, but only a cold-water flat twenty years later, the insurance company would be liable for a larger increment in later years as inflation reduced the individual's purchasing power. No financial program or annuity will insure the real value of future income or assets, and it should be recognized that this aspect of the hypothetical disability benefit program does just that. However, this protection may be exactly the kind desired by people at risk of becoming disabled. This inability of the private market to provide future benefits in real terms may be one of the strongest arguments for society-wide coverage for disability benefits.

Administration Economies of Scale

The benefit package discussed here would be very difficult to sell and administer at a reasonable cost unless a great many people purchased coverage. Lifetime coverage would mean that a company would need claims representatives wherever policyholders resided; the location and distribution of beneficiaries could be very different from the locational distribution of purchasers. Cost per claim reviewed would surely be high, unless a great many claims were handled in a particular area.

The contrast with acute health-care coverage is instructive: policies are sold to groups who make claims only within the period of purchase and who usually receive services in the same general location. Enough people have acute health care insurance, particularly Blue Cross and public insurance, so that a review of utilization and cost can cover many patients within a market area and take on a quasipublic or public character (for example, Professional Standard Review Organizations, rate-setting activities, and certificate-of-need act as utilization and cost-containment devices). Unless many beneficiaries were located in a concentrated market area, low cost, efficient administration of long-term-care benefit insurance would not be possible, and the start-up costs to reach efficient scale would surely be prohibitive.

Current Public Floor on Care

Another demand-related reason for the failure of private companies to offer disability benefit insurance is that public programs currently provide disability-related services to poor, disabled people, so that an individual can expect to purchase or be provided with at least a minimum level of care if he becomes disabled. Medicaid will only supply services after an individual expends his own income and assets. In addition, Medicaid does not provide the individual with as much choice among types of care as some private insurance plans that could be devised; specifically, institutional care is favored, congregate living arrangements are not covered, and assistance with remaining in one's own home is not covered as fully as some private policies might specify. Currently, however, every elderly citizen can be sure that, if he becomes disabled, his needs will be met at least in some minimal fashion, either at his own or public expense.

Given current public long-term-care programs, private disability benefit insurance would serve two functions that, although important, are not of quite the "life-and-death" nature of disability insurance in the absence of other coverage. The first function is protection of assets so that one need not go into poverty in the process of purchasing needed care. The second function is to provide greater choice of care, which can be built into private insurance plans. Note that greater consumer choice *could* be built into current public disability-benefit programs, at some cost. However, public programs such as public housing for the poor have typically not been oriented toward widening the consumer choice of the subsidized individuals. The demand for protection against asset loss and restriction of choice is probably less than the demand for a guarantee that, if disabled, one can receive some type of needed care. Since this second type of protection is provided by public programs, demand for private coverage is reduced.

Adverse Self-Selection

Just as people who are more likely to use health services buy more health insurance and people who are more likely to die may be expected to buy more life insurance, individuals with a higher-than-average chance of becoming disabled and/or needing more than average services if disabled would be expected to buy more disability benefit insurance. Risk assessment can be used to reduce the discrepancy between the expected value of payout for an individual and his assessed premium. Adverse selection, however, can remain a significant problem when information is poor: premium costs must rise to cover the higher-than-average benefits of high-risk people, so that more and more people with lower-than-average self-assessed risk find the insurance a "bad buy" and drop out of the program. Thus, the insurer is left covering only higher-risk people, so that premiums must rise again, causing even more relatively low-risk individuals to consider the insurance a bad buy.

The life insurance industry has designed risk-assessment techniques such as insurance physicals to identify high-risk buyers so that these buyers can be excluded or charged higher premiums concomitant with risk; group coverage by life and health insurance also works against adverse selection. Possibly, such techniques could be applied to disability benefit coverage, and adverse selection could be compensated for by screening and risk assessment. However, this information may be prohibitively expensive. The potential for adverse self-selection thus provides an argument for compulsory insurance, since when all individuals, both high and low risk, are in the covered pool, adverse self-selection is not possible.

Moral Hazard

Moral hazard is a problem endemic to all insurance, but it may be especially severe when benefits are specified as "needed services." Moral hazard is defined as a change in individual behavior induced by insurance. People are unlikely to live more dangerously knowing they have disability coverage.[3] However, disability benefit coverage (or dollar-value income-replacement coverage, for that matter) provides an incentive to overstate disability. Recovery may be influenced by the individual as well as by physical (and psychological) processes beyond his control. Moreover, disability is notoriously difficult to evaluate, and self-reporting or information from observers who may not be disinterested (for example, family and friends, providers) could bias assessed disability upward. In addition, an insurance plan under which people are provided at a zero (or low) price with what they are deemed to "need" adds incentives to provide more services than would be purchased if the insurance policy paid an equal indemnity amount and expected consumers to purchase services themselves (Pauly 1968). Because the payout is increased, premiums must be set higher than they otherwise would be, and some individuals may prefer no insurance to a policy in which they pay the expected value of more care than they would buy for themselves without insurance. Finally, when an insurance plan takes the family situation into account, the disabled insured may benefit by under-reporting his family's contribution to his care. Moral hazard for situations as difficult to assess as disability and as difficult to predict as benefit consumption may make the necessary premium for disability-expense coverage much higher than most individuals would be willing to pay (Pauly 1968).

Implications of Private Market Failure

The private market, according to our analysis, does not appear able to offer insurance for disability benefits. The most important reasons for this problem are low demand, due to the discrepancy between income and necessary premiums over the life cycle and to the "safety net" currently provided by public programs; the effect on premium price of adverse self-selection, moral hazard, and administration diseconomies; and the massive uncertainty introduced by inflation. However, it is probable that many people would be willing to pay the necessary premium or expected value of such insurance in the absence of Medicaid, and some people would be willing to pay even under current conditions in order to preserve their assets, dignity, and choice over living situation. If this proposition is accepted, it provides support for expansion of long-term-benefit coverage by public programs to insure against the risks of needing disability-related services. These risks have been specified as the risk of disability per se and the risk of being both disabled and without adequate income, family, and community resources. It should be recognized that public protection against these risks may take many forms: increased individual entitlement to care, local provision of care through single long-term-care agencies, disability payments geared to disability (parallel to indemnity insurance), expansion or reorganization of benefits through pooling of resources at a state level, and so on. By providing increased benefits to disabled people, all such programs would work to correct the current situation, in which individuals are unable to protect their ability to purchase the services they would desire for themselves if disabled. If insurance against these risks is to be provided publicly, it is necessary to consider how such an insurance program might actually be designed.

Design Issues for a Public Long-Term-Care-Insurance Program

A public program to insure against the risk of long-term-care expense must specify as clearly as any private insurance policy the following:

Which individuals are to be covered,

What risks are to be insured against and how the occurrence of insured-for events is to be determined,

What the payoff to covered individuals experiencing insured-for events will be.

Since all individuals face a risk of incurring disability-related expense, covering all United States residents under a compulsory national long-term-care-insurance seems quite reasonable. However, this discussion will focus on long-term-care-benefit insurance for people aged sixty-five and over.

The risk to be insured against is, most basically, the risk of disabling conditions expected to be of long duration. Thus, temporary disability would not trigger payment, even though the services required (posthospital nursing home care, home health visits for an acute illness) may be similar. The risk of being without family and community support may also be insurable, in the sense that higher service-benefit payoffs may be specified for disabled people without families or living situations compatible with their disabilities.

The link between the occurrence of the insured-for event (disability) and the provision of the promised benefit (service) under the insurance program is the most important design problem for a disability-expenditure-insurance program. The program must enable disabled people meeting agreed-upon criteria to consume disability-related services; but it must also ensure, for the sake of efficiency, that individuals be prevented from consuming more services than have a net benefit.[4]

Three approaches can be delineated. They differ sharply in their ability to deter such overconsumption and in their reliance on consumer and professional judgment. The first approach follows the acute health care expenditure insurance approach that covers prescribed consumption of a set of services. The second approach involves more organized need assessment by professionals and forces consideration of the cost of alternatives. The third approach allows eligible consumers to choose the amount and mix of services, with full or partial prices providing signals about the cost of various types of care.

Limits on Specific Services

Acute health care expenditure insurance is premised on the idea that people do not consume health services unless they need them, both because of the inconvenience and discomfort of services like hospitalization and because of the rationing behavior of providers. Typically, expenditures on covered services are reimbursed only up to some limit; rate setting or fee schedules limit unit cost, and peer review limits unusual amounts of care consumption. This approach could be used for long-term-care services. Only certain services would be covered, with limits on the number of days or visits. The consumer of service would simply pass his bill on to the insuring agency for payment.

The range of services currently chosen by disabled individuals should be considered for coverage under a public plan. These services include:

Nursing home care;

Care in personal care facilities;

Congregate living arrangements;

Foster care;

Day care;

Housing for the elderly;

Home health care: therapeutic, nursing, and personal care;

Chore services, homemaker services;

Meals-on-wheels;

Transportation for the handicapped;

Housing alterations necessary because of handicapping condition.

Expenditures on the program might be limited by covering only the services sought by the most severely disabled such as institutional care. The aversion of the elderly to institutional care would thus deter use of the program. Such restriction of service coverage to the most expensive types of care would have an adverse effect on efficiency, in that people would be encouraged to substitute the more costly covered service for less costly uncovered services. However, the addition of coverage of less expensive services is almost guaranteed to increase utilization and total expense, even as it lowers costs for some beneficiaries by encouraging substitution.

The service-benefit approach to health insurance is increasingly being questioned in acute care, because the gatekeepers for each service are the providers themselves, who cannot be fully disinterested rationers of care. Even more problems are likely to arise in an area where professional providers have not developed a pivotal role and where many alternative approaches differing widely in cost, may be available for a particular disability.

Determination of Needed Services

If providers and patients are likely to make consumption decisions that overutilize services, setting up a system of detailed needs assessment may be worthwhile. This system would be carried out by a disinterested gatekeeper professional or multidisciplinary team. They would specify precisely what kinds of services and how much of each type disabled individuals were eligible for. One ideal might be an objective assessment of needed services based on a disability alone; services would be paid for only if they fitted into this professionally determined least-cost treatment plan. If family and community resources are also to be taken into account, the professional assessment must go beyond an objective consideration of disabling condition alone.

This gatekeeper approach involves a number of problems. The first problem is that professional assessments of need for care based on evaluation of patients' disability are extremely variable (Sager 1979). Further, the concept of "objective" assessment of disability is muddied by the effect of the client's current environment on his degree of dependency. In addition, no strong evidence exists on the impact on health and wellbeing of various combinations of care-resource inputs to resolve disagreement on need. It would be very difficult for a long-term-care-insurance program to develop a widely acceptable set of rules stating the services to be provided for given physical conditions.

A second problem is that consumer tastes and preferences may be as important in determining outcome and quality of life for disabled people as professionals' prescription of needed services based on objective assessment of physical conditions. Long-term-care-service choices generally represent choices about day-to-day living circumstances that extend over months and years. Client satisfaction with nursing home life is likely to be greater when the individual feels he played a major role in the choice of care; this satisfaction may affect technical health-outcome measures (morbidity, mortality) as well as quality of life. It is unclear whether a gatekeeper panel charged with objectively determining the "best" set of services, given individual needs, will lead to the best outcome.[5]

A third set of assessment issues involves the relevance of family resources to benefit under the insurance program. Two alternatives are apparent. The first is to ignore the presence of a spouse, other members of the household, and family members living nearby or elsewhere and determine eligibility for services based on the individual's disabilitiy alone. This approach would mean that substantial home care would be provided to some disabled people who had family members available to assist them. On the one hand, some of these family members are not now providing needed care, so such a program would fill this gap. On the other hand, many families participate actively in the care of their elderly members, and such an alternative would substitute program payments, presumably to other workers, for care provided out of the marketplace, usually regarded as "free." Although elderly disabled people with and without family assistance would be treated alike, it is likely that those with families would be less likely to use institutional care, since family care could be added to the maximum home health benefit these people would be eligible for; equality of expenditures might lead to inequality of outcome.

The second alternative is to assess the ability of each family to provide needed assistance and to provide service entitlement only above this threshold. Under such a plan disabled people with able, but unwilling, families would be left with less care than equivalently disabled people without families. Further, if the *willingness* of families to assist was included in need assessment, by observing whether the family members were living in the same household, professing willingness to help, or not working outside the home, the logical strategy for certain families would be to encourage their disabled members to live independently, to assert unwillingness to help, or to seek market employment. Individuals whose families are unable to take these steps would, in essence, be discriminated against in the needs-assessment process and would find themselves entitled to fewer services. For example, lower-income elderly individuals are more likely to be living in the household of other family members for income reasons. If they then receive *less* assistance when disabled than people who have been able to maintain independent residences, the program would be regressive with respect to income. Likewise, there may be income correlates of mobility: middle- and upper-income families may be less likely than lower-income families to be living in close geographic proximity to elderly parents.

The problems of cost and equity involved in either alternative appear insurmountable. These problems may suggest the need for other approaches that meet needs for elderly people with and without families while minimizing the distortion of family choices introduced by public payment for long-term-care benefits. A discussion of the impact of deductible provisions for home care related to the presence of certain family members and the impact of payment to the family for services follows.

Assessment of current physical living situation might also be included in the gatekeeper approach. Some services that help disabled people function independently include transportation services and home alterations. It is inefficient to propose that someone be moved to a sheltered living arrangement, covered by insurance, because he cannot aford a relatively small expense not covered by the program to make his home more compatible with his disability, or because he is isolated by lack of transportation and community contact, also not covered. What makes more sense is to cover such services where appropriate. The ultimate outcome might be that people living in their own homes would be more likely to remain at home. People living in isolated suburban areas, without handicapped-accessible public transportation or community activities and services, might be eligible to receive more service of the social-communication-transportation type. This does not appear to be a major distribution distortion and argues for coverage of these services when they are judged to be part of a least-cost appropriate alternative.

Consumer-Choice Approach to Insurance Benefits

A third approach to determining benefit given condition would leave decisions about services to the insured consumers but would provide them with incentives to choose an efficient mix of services that maximizes benefit given cost. Such an approach would require a gatekeeper to assess the level of disability of each individual, but this assessment could be done for broad categories of disability and would not involve the prescription of specific services. The disabled individual would then be entitled to a certain level of benefit based on his level of disability and perhaps on his family and living situations. Three variations in such a program can be considered. First, the disabled insured could receive a cash payment based on his assessment, which he could spend as he saw fit. A second variation would provide consumers with a given amount of dollar-valued vouchers good only for purchase of long-term-care-services.

The disabled person with a certain dollar amount of disability benefit would have to spend it on meals-on-wheels, home health care, or nursing home care, for example, even if he could improve his situation more by increased spending on heat, food, or housing. A third variation would make the disabled individual eligible for reimbursement of expenditures on long-term-care services subject to coinsurance provisions to encourage cost consciousness.

Can Consumers Choose Services Wisely? A question that is immediately raised for any consumer-choice-oriented plan is whether disabled consumers have the ability to make wise choices about service mix and quality, especially when faced with incentives to control costs. The percentage of disabled elderly who are not competent to make such decisions may be much smaller than is commonly assumed, and the presumption of incompetency may actually increase dependency. Life satisfaction is likely to be higher when disabled people are able to have some control over their living situation and choice of support services. However, consumers should have access to advice of professionals and advocates who can supply market information since shopping for care is costly. Any consumer-choice-oriented program should thus include provision of a consumer advocate who could help consumers be more aware of their options, both when they begin entitlement to care and when a change in modality of care is considered. The advocate for each patient would inform the consumer about quality and prices of care available in that patient's market area. This information would assist in policing the market, since high-priced, low-quality services would not find buyers (unless supply is artificially restricted by other means). The consumer advocate must be the *patient's* agent, so that an advocate's placement within the administration of the long-term-care-insurance program becomes a difficult issue: if he is an employee of the government program, the agent is likely to be caught between competing goals of cost control and consumer satisfaction.

A problem might arise under the transfer-payment and voucher options if consumers spent all their resources unwisely and found themselves still in great need. The public program might still be seen as having a responsibility to "bail out" these individuals.

With respect to quality of care, suppliers of care would be encouraged to meet consumer needs and tastes under a system of free consumer choice, since consumers could (theoretically) shift modes of care if dissatisfied. However, because mobility is not great for this population, independent monitoring of service quality should be undertaken along with provision of quality information by consumer advocates. In addition, minimum standards are probably a necessity wherever care is paid for at public expense because of public feeling that, even though consumers make the choice, the government is ultimately responsible. Consumers would thus in effect be protected from the "false economy" of purchasing very inexpensive, low-quality care.

Choice among Consumer-Oriented Variations: The Case for the Copayment Option. Economists have often argued that direct transfer payments can buy more improvement in consumer welfare per dollar spent than can goverment provisions of services in kind. However, the disability payment is not likely to be politically feasible because of public concern that disabled people might spend public disability funds on goods and services not directly related to disability and that the rewards to abuse by providers would be high. Vouchers good only for disability-related services would be more appealing because of this public aversion to untied income transfers. The third consumer-oriented approach, a program that reimbursed consumers directly for long-term-care services after a coinsurance payment has been made by the consumer, might have the most leverage for cost-effective consumer decision making. Copayment can be directed against specific incentives to "overconsume" services, particularly where covered services substitute for services already purchased by the individual (housing, food) or provided by family members. In general, copayment works against the tendency to overstate disability and consume maximum services, because it reminds utilizers that services are not free.

Copayment that is proportional to the covered cost of services implies that consumers would share savings with the program if they chose the least-cost alternative and would share additional expense if they chose a mix of care that is more costly than the least-cost alternative. In addition, the bias toward institutional care, inherent in the fact that such care includes room and board, could be recognized by expecting payment from individuals of some amount representing a minimal budget for rent and food; for example, this amount could be set relative to the Supplemental Security

Income (SSI) stipend but applied to all clients, not only those receiving SSI. This room-and-board payment could be waived when the individual had to maintain a household for a spouse or was expected to return home after a relatively short institutional stay. Copayment for home care would encourage the family to supply services without payment when the opportunity cost of the caregiver's time was less than the copayment amount.

In addition, copayment can provide a method for equalizing the treatment of disabled people with and without families and for encouraging family participation in care. A deductible could be specified for home care based on the ability of the family to provide services.[6] The family's ability to provide home care would have to be judged objectively, and as noted previously, probably should not provide less service entitlement to individuals already living with their families or whose family members have already chosen nonmarket work over market work. One approach might be setting a deductible in money terms with one value if an able spouse is present, and another value (presumably lower) if any able adult children are available. Spouses and children who judged their opportunity cost of time high or adult children who lived at a distance would be expected to contribute money in place of time for the care of the disabled person. Elderly people with ungrateful or impoverished children who refused to help would suffer. The deductible would presumably be low enough so that incentives for divorce of a disabled spouse would not be strong. In many situations, the family would provide a base of support to the elderly disabled person, meeting the deductible through hours of service. The remainder of the need would be met by home care workers, subject to copayment. People without families would be eligible for more care from the program, since they would not have to meet the family deductible.

Special problems would arise if families are paid for care provided. If a family deductible and coinsurance applies, the payment to the family would be the net of these amounts. Detailed needs assessment would have to be carried out for family services, since the family would receive more money the more services they claimed to provide. Monitoring family provision of care would be a problem.

It is important to recognize in an undistorted way the value of room-and-board services provided by families when elderly members live with them. It would be ironic if a family could receive a significant amount per month for providing foster care (room, board, and minimal personal services) to an unrelated elderly individual and receive nothing for care for their own relative, who in turn could receive this service free from others. One way to avoid such distortions is to implement the room-and-board copayment for modes of care that include living arrangements; the disabled individual would thus pay some room-and-board copayment amount, plus any family deductible, for foster care with others and might be more able on this basis to persuade his family to take him in.

The preceding discussion of treatment of family resources is clearly speculative. It should serve to emphasize the need for more development of program designs that encourage undistorted resource-allocation decisions while recognizing the value of family care.

When an insurance program promises to reimburse consumers for expenditures, market prices may be greatly distorted. If prices play a role in consumer choice through deductibles and proportional coinsurance, prices will be to some extent policed by the marketplace in a way that currently does not occur. However, it may be argued that a public program should pay no more than a standard rate for each basic type of care. Public programs do not pay for the most luxurious housing, education, and food. While public programs in health care are committed to providing high-quality care for public beneficiaries, a case can be made in long-term care that additional amenities and service intensity above some standard level should not be paid for at public expense. Providers could contract to provide standard care and would accept program-determined rates as full payment for that care; or they could provide a more intensive product and be paid for the difference by the client. The second approach would lead to maximum choice both for people who prefer to pay for amenities above the standard level and for those who would rather spend their remaining income on other things. It also requires a rate-finding mechanism to set maximum prices for the standard product.

Utilization review may also be necessary to correct market imperfections. If the market operates freely, it should be profitable for providers to serve all covered people, who would be able to pay at least the resource cost of care. If monopolistic forces or external regulatory forces act to limit supply, prices may be driven up and some individuals in need may not be served. It may then be necessary to allocate available supply on the basis of level of need through utilization review of providers.

A Prototype Copayment Long-Term-Care-Insurance Plan

For the purposes of discussion it is useful to specify a prototype long-term-care-insurance plan, choosing actual coinsurance rates and specifying financing methods. The plan would allow an individual certified as disabled to select the amount and type of services he wished to make use of, subject to copayment. For clarity of presentation, only one specific form of national long-term-care insurance will be discussed here. A more complete analysis would consider the impact of the myriad policy choices available within this general option.

As discussed previously, reimbursable modes of care might be specified by needs assessment, and upper limits on reimbursement might also be set based on need, but this prototype plan relies for utilization control on the individual incentive to save resources inherent in copayment. The prototype plan treats individuals with and without families equally, rather than recognizing family availability with a deductible. An additional copayment accounting for the substitutability of institutional for home—provided room and board is added to all modes of care providing room and board in order to reduce bias toward institutionalization. The schedule of copayments is not adjusted for income, but ceilings relative to income are placed on total payment. Beneficiaries are reimbursed at standard prices for services they purchase and are permitted to supplement this reimbursement when they pay providers. This approach would be combined with some direct regulation of providers (rate setting, utilization review) and some intervention into consumer decisions by consumer advocates, since a pure market approach is unlikely to reach desired outcomes for this particular set of services and consumers. The following sections describe program dimensions in more detail.

Certification Method

Residents of the United States would be certified eligible to receive reimbursed services upon evaluation by a panel of professionals (for example, a physician, nurse, and social worker). The panel would make a yes-no decision only, based on physical dependency status. If certified for care, the individual would be reevaluated at least yearly. If the client is not certified, he could request a reevaluation after a certain time interval or after some clear change in status (for example, admission to an acute care hospital). A strong effort must be made to etablish uniform eligibility criteria across the country to reduce geographic discrepancies.

Choice of Services

The individual certified as eligible would then be able to choose among a wide range of services, after meeting a deductible. The deductible would be set to be a significant deterrent to frivolous use of the program; a figure of 10 percent of average (posttransfer) income of elderly households might be considered [for example, $300-$500 (Grad and Foster 1979)].

States could participate in the program by paying part of the deductible for needy residents; they should be discouraged from paying for all care, however, since this would end the consumers' incentive to economize. After paying the deductible in full for the first $x worth of care selected in a year, the individual would pay only a coinsurance amount for additional standard care. This coinsurance would be in two parts: first, a per diem amount reflecting the client's expected contribution to room-and/or-board costs; and second, an amount proportional to the estimated resource cost of the standard therapeutic, social, and personal care services provided in each modality. The room-and-board contribution would be a constant dollar amount for all modes that substitute for rent and/or food expense at home. It would be pegged to SSI payments, so that an individual receiving SSI would expend his expected rent and food budget if he chose institutional care; all other persons would pay this SSI budget for room and board no matter what their actual income or expenses at home. The SSI budget is not necessarily expected to cover the computed cost of nursing home, congregate housing, or foster care room-and-board services but is meant to overcome the bias toward institutionalization inherent in the *saving* of rent and food expenses for many long-term-care modes. The room-and-board copayment would be waived if the institutionalized individual had a spouse living in the community and would not be double if both spouses chose institutional care. The coinsurance for the therapeutic, nursing, and personal portions of care would be a percentage of the imputed therapeutic-nursing-personal proportions of institutional or home care prices, say, 20 percent. Consumers would be expected to pay in full for additional costs of care more luxurious or service-intensive than the recognized standard. This makes rate setting and standard setting for maximum standard care by type very important.

If incomes were adequate among the elderly, such a system of deductibles and coinsurance would not be prohibitive for anyone; the maximum spending for a person buying standard skilled nursing facility care, the most intensive care, might be $4,000 per year, not much to pay for room, board, and complete nursing care. However, this amount represents a very high proportion of income for many elderly individuals. To compensate for the low incomes of the elderly, a catastrophic ceiling on payment should be imposed, sliding with income. The ceiling might state that no one should spend more than 70 percent of income on long-term-care deductible and coinsurance payments for standard care. (Extra payment for nonstandard care would not be counted.) Once this expenditure limit has been reached, individuals would have standard care paid for in full.

What might the coinsurance look like in practice? Maximum prices would be set for each type of standard care as in the following example. Prices are presented per unit time so that costs of maintenance at home and in institutions can be compared.

Beneficiary and Program Expense for
Long-Term-Care Services under a
Prototype Insurance Program

	Price per Day	Expenditure by Consumer per Day after Meeting Deductible	Expenditure by Insurance Program per Day	Total Annual Consumer Expense with $500 Deductible
Home Care A (for example, two homemaker visits per week)	$ 5.00	$ 1.00	$ 4.00	$ 765
Home Care B (for example, two nursing visits per week)	10.00	2.00	8.00	1,130
Foster Care	12.00	7.80	4.20	3,022
Room and board	8.00	7.00		
Personal care	4.00	.80		
Intermediate Care Facility	20.00	9.00	11.00	3,560
Room and board	10.00	7.00		
Personal, therapeutic care	10.00	2.00		
Skilled Nursing Facility Care	35.00	10.00	25.00	4,007
Room and board	10.00	7.00		
Personal, therapeutic care	15.00	3.00		

In the example presented in the table, the consumer pays 20 percent of the cost of standard personal, therapeutic, and social service care, plus a flat $7 per day for all options including room and board, no matter what the actual cost of providing these services is in different settings. Of course, the individual pays the full price until the deductible ($500) is met, buying 100 days of maintenance through home care at $5, or 50 days at $10, or 25 days of ICF care at $20, and so on. The far right hand column of the example shows the maximum yearly payment.

An upper limit would be set on the per diem program payment for home care services, so that consumers would be encouraged to shift to institutional care whenever it is overwhelmingly more efficient.

Payment to family members for services to elderly relatives is an especially difficult issue. If family care can be treated as substitutes for home care agencies and foster care with similar supervision and monitoring requirements, it would be wise to pay them on the same basis. The disabled individual would still be expected to pay the deductible and coinsurance, but this requirement might be met through family service. An alternative might be to pay families at a lower rate, but also to provide them with free (in-kind) support like respite care for a certain number of weeks per year or a given number of hours per week.

Finance

The program could be financed in a number of ways. All the finance options available for acute care national health insurance could be considered (CBO 1977; Davis 1975). However, a combined public-private approach with standard benefit packages purchased from private insurers is probably ruled out for all the reasons, discussed previously, that the private provision of disability *benefit* insurance has proved unwieldy. (Note that a public program would not *replace* private coverage because it is very minimal, and therefore public provision and financing should be more politically acceptable.)

Several alternatives for public financing of the program could be considered. Since coverage would be equal for all residents, an argument could be made for equal yearly payments from all individuals over a certain age, making the program equivalent to a compulsory community-rated lifetime-payment disability-benefit plan that might be offered on the private market. The actuarially necessary premium payments would be a much larger proportion of annual income for poor people than for people with higher incomes. Such a regressive form of finance (equivalent to a head tax) is not politically appealing, and a financing mode that is progressive with respect to income would probably be more attractive. A second alternative is payroll tax finance, in which individuals would purchase equal coverage by payment proportional to wage and salary income. This alternative would tend to be regressive taxation as well (although milder than the flat head tax) because higher income people receive more income from nonwage sources. A third alternative—sharing financing with states—would again inject a regressive element into the finance mechanism, since states tend to levy sales taxes and property taxes that are regressive with income. (Since the program would replace Medicaid, *avoiding* state finance would mean windfall budget gains for states that have heavily supported Medicaid long-term-care services.)

A fourth public approach is finance through general revenues. Analyses of financing methods for national health insurance have supported this method (CBO 1977). This approach would cause a transfer of resources from current income earners to the currently covered population and, more specifically, to those receiving benefits. Like our Social Security system, it would result in an intergenerational transfer of resources. Is such a program "insurance"? Yes, in the same way that national health insurance plans are insurance: current income earners face a risk of needing benefits and by maintaining the program are providing for their own coverage.

Predicting Impacts of a National Long-Term-Care-Insurance Program

What Effects Are Important?

Several goals often espoused for health policy change, specifically cost containment, enhancement of the access to care of the population with health needs, and maintenance or improvement of quality of care, can be seen as subsumed in a broader framework of public willingness to pay for a given benefit distribution. On the one hand are increased benefits: more care for some individuals, and higher-quality care for others, producing an improvement in health outcome and quality of life for the covered population. The access and quality goals focus on these benefits. On the other hand are increased costs: the increased amounts of resources, public and private, that would flow into care for disabled people. Consideration of any particular policy change in this net benefit framework requires first that the amount and distribution of changes in utilization be considered, with attention also to changes in quality of care; and second, that the amount and distribution of cost increases be projected. Also important to consider are aspects of a proposed program that affect its political and administrative feasibility. These aspects include the program's probable effect on provider groups, its administrative complexity, and in a larger sense, its underlying policy approach, termed here its *policy values*. The aspects of the long-term-care-benefit-insurance program proposed here are considered in turn in the next sections for comparability with other long-term-care options in this volume. This evaluation framework raises many questions that are difficult to answer with current information; therefore, the chapter concludes with a call for research that is needed before such a program proposal can be reasonably evaluated.

Distribution of Benefits Under Long-Term-Care Insurance: Who Would Receive More or Less Care?

A national long-term-care-insurance program would change the amount and type of care provided for many groups of individuals. These increments and decrements to utilization should be examined by disability status, income, family situation, and location, because increased benefits to each group may be valued differently.

One way to approach this problem is to categorize people along these four dimensions and project utilization for each group. For example, high-disability individuals with high incomes and no family support are probably currently making use of needed institutional care and home support services no matter where they live; coverage through national long-term-care insurance might marginally increase utilization, since the relative price of purchased care would fall. Because this group is already using services to a great extent, large changes in utilization are unlikely. High-income people in rural areas might not be receiving the care they need because of lack of service capacity; an increase in demand from middle-income and poor people would be expected to induce an expansion in supply in areas where service provision has not been profitable, so that people not receiving care only because of lack of supply could then receive it. Similar arguments might be made for each group to arrive at predictions about increased utilization or change in mode of care.

This analysis may be generalized by realizing that current utilization by an individual is the result of a demand relationship, where the quantity (Q) of care of a given type demanded by disabled individuals is a function of:

Health status (Q increases with disability);

Income (Q increases with income);

Out-of-pocket price of care (Q decreases as price rises; price for some services is lowered by Medicaid eligibility, available to people with low incomes, and varying by state);

Relative prices of substitute services (Q increases with price of substitutes);

Availability of family support (Q decreases with increased availability of family support: less home care is purchased, given price, and the probability of institutionalization is less, ceteris paribus, if family is present).

The national long-term-care-insurance plan changes two variables in this relationship. First, the out-of-pocket *price of care* to people not covered by Medicaid falls, and the price to people currently covered rises, since they must now make copayments for services. Second, the *relative price* of institutional services rises in comparison to the price of home care services (while both prices fall absolutely). These changes occur because the copayment for services including room and board includes a flat rate in addition to a copayment proportional to therapeutic and personal care costs.

The first effect should increase utilization of all services. Since poor people (currently covered by Medicaid) would probably have their deductible reduced and would quickly reach the income-related payment ceiling, the price increase to them would not be very meaningful. Increases in service utilization would be largest for groups with strong reasons to use care (high disability, lack of family) for whom price has been a real barrier;

middle- and lower-middle-income disabled, especially those without family, probably fall into this category.

The changes in relative prices for institutional and noninstitutional care should shift utilization from nursing homes to home care even as total utilization is growing. This shift should be especially strong for the Medicaid group, which currently faces a low price for nursing home care and faces full-market price for uncovered home services. (In addition, covered home services are often not available because of low supply; care is likely to be more widely available after a demand increase if there are local economies of scale).

While the amount of purchased care would be likely to increase for all groups, family-provided care would still be attractively inexpensive for many people with families, especially retired spouses. Thus the increase in purchased service should be less for people with families than for those without, and families would still be encouraged to provide care for disabled relatives. Because the disabled family member would be eligible for home care regardless of family status, we might even expect to see *more* family-provided care: rather than facing an all-or-nothing decision between complete family care and institutionalization, the family and the disabled member could arrive at a mix, in which family care and purchased home care or day care were both provided. If care by family members is deemed especially valuable, a policy of paying for family care could encourage this. The family deductible discussed in the broad consideration of insurance against loss of family is not included in this prototype program. Such a deductible could encourage family-provided care by raising the price of alternatives to disabled people with families, thus making the relative price of family care even lower.

Utilization may currently be less than demand for some groups because of supply restrictions. If supply remains limited, it is conceivable that much of the increase in demand for care by type would remain unrealized. This assumption underlies the CBO projections for long-term-care expenditures under universal long-term-care insurance for the elderly: it was assumed that supply could not respond instantaneously, and therefore that initial growth of utilization, and thus expenditures, would be minimal (CBO, 1977). The insurance option as described here does not rely on direct supply restriction (specifically certificate-of-need) to curtail utilization. Possibly, however, rates paid to providers for care would not be set high enough to elicit new supply. Rationing devices like utilization review at the provider level could be called into play to encourage providers to serve the most disabled despite limited supply.

Quality of Care

The specified insurance option includes provision for monitoring the quality of care of particular providers, both through direct regulation and through better-informed consumer choice among providers. When the consumer takes an active role and is actually assisted in "voting with his feet" against low-quality providers, quality of care can be policed by consumers and abuse of patients avoided: they are not a captive population. In addition, consumers with the advice of advocates would be making choices among care alternatives that fit their individual tastes and circumstances. Individuals have been shown to do better in nursing homes when the choice of facility and the choice to enter an institution was their own; this impact on outcome is likely to hold over the broad spectrum of care. While consumers may not always choose what professionals would select as "best," still the best way to maximize consumer satisfaction and quality of life is apparently for individuals to make their own choices, subject to appropriate resource constraints.

Continuity of care, including acute health care and all long-term-care modalities, may also have an effect on overall outcome for disabled people and is certainly a relevant aspect of quality of care. Continuity is not stressed by this prototype insurance program, except insofar as it can be encouraged by better-informed patients and by advocates' or agents' serving them. One can envision provisions, however, allowing individuals to combine their entitlements to acute health care and long-term-care coverage to buy into an organization providing comprehensive care, for example, a social/health maintenance organization, which would supply desirable continuity.

Cost of the Program

The total cost to public and private budgets of the insurance option is difficult to assess without good demand estimates of the impact of absolute and relative price changes and on utilization by mode of care. The federal government would certainly not be paying all current long-term-care expenditures, because individuals would be expected to meet deductibles and pay coinsurance and would pay privately for care beyond a specified standard. Thus private payment for care would still be large, especially since relatively well-off people might be encouraged to use the government payment as a base to purchase high-amenity care. The shift in relative prices encouraging less institutionalization would be unlikely actually to reduce institutional care, since apparently significant numbers of people living at home are in need of institutional care. When this care becomes less expensive to them, they may well enter nursing homes (Berg et al. 1970). However, many people who would have sought institutional care in the past will now have other more attractive alternatives including home care, day care, and other home support services. Thus, less institutional care would be provided than under an equivalent insurance program funding only institutional care.

The amount of home care sought by people now managing on their own, perhaps with family and community support, is likely to be large. The belief is strong among professionals and other observers that such home support can defer institutionalization, prolong life, and increase quality of life; more important from the point of view of insurance, it is what disabled individuals want for themselves. Thus many people, both disabled and not, young and old, would want to insure for home care services if they could. The disabled elderly are currently deterred from consuming home care by price barriers and inadequate supply. While the cost of this aspect of the insurance option would be great, if taxpayers can view it as setting a program in motion that will protect their own ability to purchase needed and desired home services when they become elderly and disabled, we should be willing to pay as a society for such a high-benefit program.

Effects on Providers

Somewhat contrary to the net-benefit framework is to take a separate view of the insurance option from a provider perspective. Evaluation of net benefit focuses on increased benefits to disabled people and their families and on costs borne by them and by taxpayers; double counting resource inputs and outputs by considering also the revenue losses and gains to providers is incorrect. However, resources do not always shift as freely as classic cost-benefit analysis assumes. This factor may justify attention to which types of providers would be helped or hurt by a new long-term-care-insurance program. Utilization shifts have been discussed previously; the most salient shifts would be increases in home care and decreases in some institutional care. Providers would be expected to respond to these shifts in demand, just as other producers in the economy respond to demand shifts; the growth of nursing homes would be slowed, and resources would flow into the home care sector. Regulation of providers' rates and quality would continue; some utilization review would also be put in place to assure that care is going to the most needy.

Administrative Complexity and Expense

The insurance option, relying as it does on decentralized decision making by consumers, does not require an elaborate decision-making organization to approve every change in utilization as appropriate, or to deny care as unneeded. A mechanism must be developed to approve patients for entrance into the program but detailed needs assessment would not be required. Regulation of rates and quality would continue to be administratively difficult but would not be greatly changed from current practice. The consumer advocates, who would provide information and assistance to patients making choices about initiating care or changing mode of care, would have to function independently of regulators and budgetary authorities if they were to represent patients' interest, and this may be difficult to achieve administratively.

Policy Values

The key value stressed in the national long-term-care-insurance program as specified here is consumer choice: the idea that the consumer has the best understanding of his tastes and his own situation, and if provided with access to long-term-care resources and good information, can make decisions about care that will maximize his own quality of life. If consumer choice is valued by policymakers, this approach is to be preferred over precise specification of needed care by professionals, who may maximize appropriateness of health care in a technical sense but may not fully take into account the patients' tastes and self-perceived needs.

Research Needs

Consideration of a prototype national long-term-care-insurance program suggests two major related directions for future research before a plan can actually be fully specified. First is a better analysis of demand for long-term care by modality, concentrating on the variables in the demand function (own price and prices of substitutes) that would be altered by various parameters in a long-term-care-insurance program.

Second, either using estimated demand elasticities from this research or simulating over a range of elasticity values, it would be worthwhile to simulate the impact of various deductible and coinsurance provisions, income-related ceilings on total payment, and treatment of family inputs. Simulation has provided instructive results for national acute care health insurance (Feldstein et al. 1972), and while the initial data necessary for simulating individual behavior will not be as straightforward to obtain, the feasibility of such a simulation should be investigated.

Notes

1. An example may be helpful to those unaccustomed to thinking of insurance in this generic fashion. If there is a 0.1 percent chance of a totally destructive fire in a factory valued at a million dollars, the owner would be interested in paying some relatively small amount to protect his investment.

If the insurance company is insuring many such buildings, it will be willing to sell him the contingent claim stating "Pay one million dollars if the factory burns down" for a price of 0.1 percent × $1,000,000, plus an allowance for administrative expenses and profit, or just over $1,000. A risk-averse individual would probably be willing to pay a good deal more than this, even $2,000 or $3,000, to be certain of avoiding such a large loss.

2. A third type of insurance might set a money payoff that would directly compensate for the disability. For example, if Mr. Jones becomes paralyzed, he would receive $x to replace income he loses from the inability to work at his former job, $y to pay for personal care and rehabilitation services that allow him to reach his highest possible level of function, and compensatory damages of $z, say $1 million a year, that in essence make him feel as well off as he was before his disablement. This third type of payoff is not considered here, but see Zeckhauser (1973).

3. The classic moral-hazard situation would be one in which a driver with vandalism insurance parks in riskier areas than the uninsured or a factory owner with fire insurance is more careless with combustible materials.

4. Pauly's concept of "unnecessary" surgery, operations for which cost exceeds what a fully informed consumer would pay, is useful here (Pauly 1979).

5. See Sager (1979, pp. 110-124) for a review of the literature on consumer choice in long-term care.

6. Two potential reasons for encouraging family-service provisions should be distinguished. The first is that family services appear free to the government and reduce public budgets. However, treating family labor as free distorts resource allocation decisions. For example, the woman who is forced to give up a highly skilled job to care for an aged parent replaces highly valued productive activity with less valued production, which could be supplied in part by less skilled workers. This is inefficient, and lowers society's total production of goods and services below its potential level.

The second reason for valuing family care is that family participation in personal care of elderly disabled people is an expression of family strength and social values. According to such reasoning, society should be willing to pay the daughter *more* to care for her parent than it is willing to pay an outsider. However, some would argue that any payment to relatives undermines the philanthropic nature of the gift relationship. Lip service is given to the value of nonmarket work (volunteer work, child rearing, and home making, as well as care for disabled family members), but those who choose such uses for their time in spite of significant opportunity cost are generally not rewarded with the benefits accompanying market employment (for example, Social Security coverage, pensions, and health insurance, as well as money wages). More analysis of family decisions and of social values is needed before these issues can be fully explored. See Callahan et al. (1980) for background on these issues.

References

Arrow, K.J. 1963. "Uncertainty and the Welfare Economics of Medical Care." *American Economic Review* 53:5 (December):941-973.

Berg, R.L., Browning, F.E., Hill, J.G., and Senkert, W. 1970. "Assessing the Health Needs of the Aged." *Health Services Research* 5:1 (Spring): 36-59.

Callahan, Jr., J.J., Diamond, L.D., Giele, J.Z., and Morris, R. 1980. "Responsibility of Families for their Severely Disabled Elders." *Health Care Financing Review* 1:3 (Winter):29-48.

Congressional Budget Office, U.S. Congress. 1977. *Long-Term Care for the Elderly and Disabled.* Washington, D.C.: Government Printing Office.

Davis, K. 1975. *National Health Insurance: Benefits, Costs and Consequences.* Washington, D.C.: Brookings Institution.

Feder, J., and Holahan, J. 1979. *Financing Health Care for the Elderly: Medicare, Medicaid, and Private Health Insurance.* Washington, D.C.: Urban Institute.

Feldstein, M., Friedman, B., and Luft, H. 1972. "Distributional Aspects of National Health Insurance Benefits and Finance." *National Tax Journal* XXV:4 (December):497-510

Grad, S., and Foster, K. 1979. *Income of the Population 55 and Over, 1976.* U.S. Department of Health, Education, and Welfare, Social Security Administration, SSA Pub. No. 13-11865. Washington, D.C.: Government Printing Office.

Kastenbaum, R., and Candy, S.E. 1973. "The Four Percent Fallacy." *Aging and Human Development* 4:1 (Winter):15-21.

Mitchell, M.B., and Schwartz, W.B. 1976. "The Financing of National Health Insurance." *Science* 192:4,240 (May 14):621-629.

Palmore, E. 1976. "Total Chance of Institutionalization Among the Aged." *The Gerontologist* 16:6 (December):504-507.

Pauly, M.V. 1968. "The Economics of Moral Hazard." *American Economic Review* 85:3 (June):531-537.

_____. 1979. "What is Unnecessary Surgery?" *Health and Society* 57:1 (Winter):195-217.

Sager, A. 1979. *Learning the Home Care Needs of the Elderly: Patient, Family, and Professional Views of an Alternative to Institutionalization.* Final Report, AOA Grant 90-A-1026. Levinson Policy Institute, Brandeis University.

Zeckhauser, R.J. 1973. "Coverage for Catastrophic Illness." *Public Policy* 21:2 (Spring):149-172.

5 Disability Allowance for Long-Term Care

Leonard W. Gruenberg
and *Karl A. Pillemer*

Professionals are in agreement that a substantial portion of elderly persons are institutionalized, not because they are in need of skilled nursing care but because they require some degree of supervision and aid with personal care or household maintenance activities in order to live at home (Davis and Gibbon 1971; Frohlich 1971; Nash 1966; Pettigrew and Kinloch 1971; Williams et al. 1973). These individuals do not have family available and willing to provide such assistance and/or they lack the economic resources with which to purchase those services. Cash or in-kind benefits based on disability levels may help the impaired elderly to avoid (or at least to postpone) costly nursing home placement. In this report, a number of alternative variations of a disability payment program are put forward, and a preliminary analysis of those variations is presented.

A disability payment program may be regarded as one possible variant of a long-term-care-insurance program and was discussed in this context by Bishop in chapter 4. In practice, however, such a program would of necessity be of narrower scope than a full long-term-care-insurance program. Design problems discussed later in this chapter would limit the program so that it could provide cash payments or vouchers to individuals who can continue to reside in the community but who need assistance in the activities of daily living (for example, bathing, dressing) and/or homemaker, chore, and companionship services. It could not be expected to pay for visiting nurse service, skilled nursing home care or other more medically oriented services. Because of this difference, major program design issues are different than the issues that need to be considered in examining a broad ranged long-term-care-insurance program. For this reason the disability allowance as a long-term-care option is being given a separate treatment in this chapter. Two previous treatments of this option, however, are summarized by Youket in the appendix to this volume (Pollak 1976; Correia 1976).

The first section of the chapter presents a brief statement of the problem. Next, certain key issues in the design of a disability allowance are discussed, including eligibility requirements and the question of the method

The authors are grateful to Janet Mitchell for offering her considerable insights into the complex issues that need to be resolved before a successful disability allowance program can be developed. Thanks are also due to Robert Morris for his invaluable critical comments.

and level of payment. The importance of informal supports is analyzed as well as the issues revolving around the choice of a cash payment or a voucher system. Finally, the experience of other nations using a disability allowance is reviewed.

The second section of the chapter evaluates the effect of this option on providers, consumers, and the delivery of services. The relative advantages and disadvantages of a program of this kind are considered in relation to other long-term-care options.

Statement of the Problem

The disabled historically have been eligible for transfer payments under two separate public programs: Old Age, Survivors, Disability and Health Insurance (OASDHI) and Aid to the Permanently and Totally Disabled (APTD).[1] These payments are designed only to protect against lost earnings due to disability and not to meet any special needs that may arise as a result. The disability insurance portion of OASDHI was legislated in 1956 and is subject to similar eligibility and benefit formulas as old-age pensions under Social Security. In addition, the recipient must be unable to work as the result of permanent disability. Thus, a disability pension is an entitlement for the disabled worker who has contributed for a sufficient period to the Social Security program. APTD is a public-welfare program dating back to 1935 for persons who are not only permanently disabled but also poor. In 1974 this program, along with two other categorical assistance programs (Old Age Assistance and Aid to the Blind), were replaced by SSI, and uniform eligibility requirements and benefit levels were established. The potential recipient must still qualify as one of the "worthy poor;" he must be old, blind, or completely disabled, and he must meet both an income and assets test. Benefits are reduced by the amounts of any income except for small amounts of earned income that are disregarded.

The historical precedent for special benefits for the disabled is clear. The issue of selecting an entitlement program or a means-tested program (for instance, special insurance versus public relief), however, is not. Examination of health insurance benefits for the disabled reveals the same dichotomy. Social Security beneficiaries of old-age pensions (including the disabled elderly) and of some disability pensions (primarily end stage renal disease patients) are eligible for Medicare. SSI recipients, on the other hand, qualify for a welfare medical program, Medicaid, although the poor elderly will often receive health-care benefits under both programs.

Issues in Disability Allowance Program Design

The development of a supplemental benefits program to encourage disabled persons to remain at home could resemble either an insurance program such as Medicare or a public assistance program like Medicaid. Before designing such a disability program, several major issues need to be resolved.

Eligibility Requirements: How should disability be defined for eligibility purposes? Should the program be restricted to any particular age groups? Should eligibility and/or benefit levels vary as a function of family support? Should eligibility for benefits depend solely on the presence of disability, or should applicants also meet a means test? Should payments be made only to individuals who reside in their own or their family's home, or should they also be made to individuals who reside in foster care homes, other types of domiciliary care homes, or in long-term-care institutions?

Payment Structure: Should a single level of payment be involved or several levels depending on the extent of disability? In the latter case should the payment level be based upon the cost of services not generally covered under existing programs (for instance, homemaker and attendant care) or should it be based upon a much wider range of long-term-care services including medical care? Should the payment levels be dependent upon the availability of family support? Should they be dependent on individual or upon family income?

Method of Payment: What is the preferred—that is, socially optimal— means of transfer? Should benefits be made in cash to the consumer who then purchases the necessary services? Or should more restricted grants be provided, for example, in the form of vouchers earmarked for a specified set of services?

Each of these issues—eligibility requirements, payment structure, and method of payment—is discussed in the following sections.

Eligibility Requirements

Disability. The definition of disability for eligibility purposes depends largely upon policy objectives. Since Social Security disability pensions have an earnings replacement function, the inability to work as a result of disease or injury is the critical criterion. For a target population that has already withdrawn from the labor force, this definition is clearly not appropriate. As discussed before, the absence of social and economic supports at home, rather than the need for skilled nursing care, may lead to nursing home admission. A reasonable policy objective might be to reduce unnecessary institutionalization by providing (or making available) those supports to individuals who require them.

Given this objective, eligibility might be determined by functional incapacity and the resulting need for physical assistance from another individual. Under this definition disability, as defined by some insurance programs, is a necessary but insufficient condition for eligibility. Some mildly disabled persons, and even persons considered by some standards to be severely disabled, might not be eligible for benefits unless they also require the physical assistance of another person. In contrast to this concept, under some disability programs (for example, the Veteran's Administration, Workmen's Compensation) both pensions and attendant allowances have been awarded based on the percent of total disability with different weights assigned to the loss or incapacity of different body parts. A blind person with only one arm might, for example, be deemed 50 percent disabled under these programs. This definition of disability may be an appropriate one to use for those insurance programs whose benefits are intended to replace lost income. However, with a cane or a dog, this disabled person might be fully mobile and able to care for himself. Thus, in the absence of some other handicapping condition that restricted self-care activities, this person would not be eligible for benefits under the proposed program. The proposed definition of disability—uncompensated impairment and the resulting functional incapacity leading to the need for assistance from another individual—has the obvious advantage of tying eligibility directly to the need for services.

Eligibility might also be restricted to cases of permanent disability, excluding persons with short-term-disabling conditions who are expected to resume their normal activities (for example, convalescence and rehabilitation following a fractured hip). These individuals would continue to be eligible for extended-care benefits under other public programs. Permanent disability would include chronic handicapping disorders such as arthritis, congestive heart failure, and so on (irreversible conditions that are expected to worsen with time). The permanently disabled are among those most at risk of institutionalization. Constant attendant allowances for the permanently disabled have been implemented by twenty-seven countries—all of the industrialized and Western European countries except Canada, West Germany, and the United States—precisely for this reason (Tracy 1974).

Age. Eligibility for program benefits could be limited to those individuals aged 65 and over, or the program could also include younger persons (for instance, individuals in the age group 18-64). Although the disability prevalence rate increases with age, a comparable number of persons under and over 65 have significant functional impairments. In fact, the National Center for Health Statistics estimates that more than 6.9 million persons, 17 years of age and older, are unable to carry out their majority activity (Wilder 1977). Forty-nine percent or 4 million persons are under the age of 65. These statistics suggest that a disability payment program should be directed towards adults of all ages.

However, although disability can be observed among all age groups, the likelihood of a person's becoming permanently institutionalized increases with age much more rapidly than does the prevalence rate of disability. Thus, for example, the National Center for Health Statistics reports that nearly 9 of every 10 persons in nursing homes are over 65 (National Center for Health Statistics 1979). A major reason for this out-of-proportion rate of institutionalization among elderly persons is the increasing likelihood, as a person gets older, that he or she will not have an available family member who can help to provide care in the event that illness and disability should occur.

If the main objective of the disability payment program is to prevent avoidable institutionalization, a reasonable strategy would thus be to limit eligibility to elderly persons, at least during the test phase of such a program, although the authors of this chapter believe that in the long run establishing such a program on an age-integrated basis would be desirable. The discussions in the following sections assume that program eligibility will be limited to elderly persons.

Family Status. Eligibility and/or benefit levels could be tied to the existence of certain family members who could provide support, including spouse and/or children. It is known that a substantial proportion of support services to the elderly are provided informally by family members. Elderly persons without these supports—that is, those who live alone and/or do not have children residing nearby—are more at risk of institutionalization than those having social supports. If the policy objective is to avoid unnecessary nursing home placement, this group should be the logical target population for special long-term-care benefits. The family-attached elderly could be excluded from the program altogether or be eligible for lower benefit levels. This approach would reduce the substitution of public care for private family care and focus scarce dollars on those most in need. However, two major drawbacks exist. First, to the extent that family members are a proxy for greater economic resources, this approach resembles a means test that in itself has certain drawbacks. (This issue is discussed in detail in a later section). Second, there would be an incentive on the part of the spouse or children to abandon the disabled applicant. We have already witnessed this phenomenon in another program predicated (in part) on the primacy of family responsibility: AFDC.

Payment Structure

Under an alternative approach, both eligibility and payment levels would be independent of family status. All disabled persons would benefit from such a program, although those with families would clearly be better off. Families are notably more efficient in the production of health than are single persons (Grossman 1972). Recipients with families would have more inputs (both purchased and family-provided services) necessary to attain a desirable level of health as well as greater flexibility in combining these inputs.

The single individual presumably would need to purchase all personal care services using income supplemented by the disability allowance; if the price of these necessary services exceeded his ability to pay, he would eventually be forced to substitute institutional for noninstitutional care. The question of whether the disability payments should continue when the individual enters an institution is discussed later. The family-attached elderly person could use his disability payment to obtain services in addition to those provided gratis by relatives. The disability benefits could be used to supplement family care in a variety of ways. For example, the disability benefits might be used to obtain part-time attendant care for an individual who requires around-the-clock observation. Family members might be unable to provide twenty-four-hour services over a period of years, months, or even weeks. Emotional bankruptcy and physical exhaustion could force an otherwise caring family to institutionalize a disabled relative. This undesirable outcome would thus be prevented or delayed by the disability allowance.

As a second example, family members might choose to remain at home and provide additional care rather than enter the labor market, if they could be at least partially reimbursed for the services they provide. Alternatively, family members with high productivity in market activities might choose to substitute homemaker or attendant services for their own time. Some evidence already exists that this substitution is occurring with regard to institutional care. The labor force participation rate of adult married women has been shown to significantly raise the demand for nursing home care (Chiswick 1976). Making disability payments to elderly who are part of these working families could enable some of these families to maintain their elderly parents at home for a longer time.

A recent study by Sussman (1979) provides support for the argument that disability payments should be made to individuals with family support as well as to those without. A sample of residents of Cleveland, Ohio, and Winston-Salem, North Carolina, were asked to rank their preference for three programs that would be made available to help them support an old person in their family's home. The choices were a monthly check, food stamps, or a tax deduction. The overwhelming majority indicated that the monthly check would aid them in caring for an elderly relative, citing the flexibility of that option. Sussman cautions, however, that most respondents reported some willingness to take in an elderly relative regardless of the support program and that the program should perhaps be viewed as an additional reinforcement to that predisposition.

Taking all of these factors into account, a reasonable resolution would be to tie the level of payments, but not the eligibility for benefits, to the presence or absence of a spouse and of children. This idea is discussed in more detail by Bishop in chapter 4.

Income and Assets. A key eligibility issue for policy purposes is whether all disabled persons should qualify for benefits, regardless of income and/or assets, or whether they should be required to pass a means test. Under one form of means-tested program, disabled individuals whose family income and/or assets exceed a predetermined level would not receive any benefits. They must spend down to this amount before becoming eligible for payment. Eligibility for both Medicaid and SSI is based on this type of formula. Alternatively, benefits could be set based on an income-related sliding scale. Poorer persons would be eligibile for relatively large payments with the size of the benefits diminishing as income rose. The food stamp program operates on a sliding scale, albeit within a narrow range.

For eligibility purposes, family income might be defined as disposable income for all sources (both earned and unearned) for the individual and his or her spouse if married. Alternatively, policymakers might want to include the incomes of adult children when assessing the eligibility of disabled parents. Ceteris paribus, this inclusion would result in a redistribution of benefits away from recipients with families to the unattached elderly, a group presumably at greater risk for institutionalization. As discussed earlier, however, holding children financially liable for their parents' care may result in an abdication of their responsibilities. Also, as was recently pointed out by Callahan et al. (1980), a means test applied to family members not living in the household would be likely to arouse serious opposition and tests in the courts. All other things being equal, a means-tested program has one major advantage over programs not tied to income or wealth: it would be less costly. Limiting the pool of eligible recipients would result in lower total program expenditures. Disabled individuals would be forced to first use their own income and/or assets to obtain needed services before they could qualify for benefits. An income-related disability program has at least four drawbacks, however. First, and most important, disabled persons with incomes only slightly above this level (the near poor) would be precluded from receiving any benefits whatsoever, while individuals with incomes only marginally lower would be entitled to the full range of benefits. This might have the perverse effect of encouraging the near poor to enter nursing homes where they could rapidly spend down to the required income level. An income-related sliding scale could minimize the negative effects, however. Second, the stigma attached to a means-tested program may discourage needy individuals from applying for benefits. This stigma is allegedly a problem with the SSI program. Third, the administrative structure required to assess income eligibility would increase costs and limit the cost savings mentioned. Fourth, programs designed solely for the poor (for example, Medicaid) may have less political appeal, and if approved, are apt to be chronically underfunded (Davis and Reynolds 1976).

In the absence of a means test for determining eligibiliy or for determining the size of the copayment (if an income-related sliding-fee scale is adopted), benefits would become a universal entitlement based on disability alone. This entitlement would explicitly recognize the special needs of the disabled and remove the stigma of welfare.

The question of whether an individual and his or her family will have to meet an assets test as well must be considered. If such a test is required, certain assets might be excluded, such as a residence occupied by the recipient. Under the SSI program, for example, applicants must first meet an assets test, and then benefits are reduced as income increases. Several forms of assets are excluded, however, including a home and various types of income-producing property. Issues such as these deserve a more detailed analysis than is possible here and would have to be resolved before the proposed plan could be put in effect.

Living Arrangements. If the policy objective of a disability allowance is to encourage community living for the disabled elderly, payments might be made only to individuals not living in institutions. Alternatively, policymakers might want to maximize consumer choice and allow the benefits to be utilized by individuals who need or who choose to live in an institutional setting as well. An intermediate approach might be to extend payments only for individuals living in sheltered living arrangements other than nursing homes, including foster homes, personal care homes, and other types of domiciliary care facilities, as well as sheltered housing units. This would stimulate the supply of those settings relative to nursing homes.

Allowing beneficiaries to apply their disability allowance payments toward nursing home care would have a major advantage. Together with their pensions, many individuals would be able to purchase care as private rather than Medicaid patients. Consumers may then be encouraged to shop for low-priced, high-quality care. To the extent that such shopping did occur, competition would be stimulated in the nursing home industry.

Domiciliary care facilities primarily are intended to provide sheltered living arrangements and personal care to individuals who do not need around-the-clock medical or nursing care but who, because of reduced functional capacity and inadequate informal support, are unable to live independently in the community. Providing individuals who choose this type of living arrangement with a disability allowance would be quite appropriate—in fact, a similar type of payment system to individuals is currently in operation in some states that have chosen to supplement SSI payments for individuals in domiciliary care.

Number of Distinct Payment Levels. A single level of payment could go to all eligible individuals whose level of disability exceeded a certain threshold.

Alternatively, several payment levels based upon the level of disability of the individual could be used. The multiple-payment system would be more efficient economically, since it would target payments more precisely to the level of need than the single-payment system. However, the multiple-payment system would require more detailed assessments and would hence require a more complex and expensive administrative structure. Nonetheless, the multiple-payment system would appear to be more desirable.

Basis for Determining Level of Payment. The level of payment to a disabled individual should be based upon an estimate of the costs of services the individual needs as a result of his disability. The issue to be decided is the range of services to be included in making this estimate. Presumably, the benefit levels could be set high enough to include payment for medical, skilled nursing, and other health care services currently covered by Medicare and Medicaid. It is argued later, however, that the level of payment be figured on the basis of a more limited set of sevices—those long-term-care services that either are not covered services under other programs or are inadequately provided. This type would probably include the following services: personal care—assistance with activities or daily living such as bathing, mobility, and so on; and homemaker and chore services—assistance with household maintenance activities such as cooking, shopping, cleaning, and so on.

The inclusion of this set of services under a disability allowance program has several advantages. First, the absence of such supportive services are frequently cited as the primary reasons for nursing home admissions. The availability of these services presumably would help prevent future deteriorations in health and allow many disabled recipients to remain at home.

Second, medical and skilled nursing services are more generally available for the elderly. Medicare beneficiaries are entitled to unlimited physician visits annually.[2] Nonmedical long-term-care services, however, are usually either not available or not adequate to meet the needs of a disabled population. While personal care services are included in the home health service benefits package, they are restricted to the two-hundred-visit maximum. Although this maximum may be appropriate for nursing and other skilled services, it may not be adequate for personal care services that may be required on a daily basis or for several hours or more at a time. Homemaker and chore services, furthermore, are specifically excluded under Medicare. Some state Medicaid programs do provide personal care and homemaker services, but these services are limited by eligibility requirements, benefit ceilings, and the vicissitudes of state politics. Title XX programs are similarly limited in terms of population served and scope of benefits.

Third, estimates of the need for personal care services could very likely be tied directly to numerical indexes used to measure disability levels without necessitating the development of a complex case management approach, thus reducing the administrative costs of the program. Service needs would be relatively stable and hence predictable over longer periods of time, which would facilitate program planning and eliminate the need for frequent reassessments. Wide variation in medical and skilled nursing needs across and within disability levels probably would require a more case-specific approach such as that currently used by Medicare. (The physician in this instance must both certify the need for care and prescribe the type and amount of services required.) These latter services are also less predictable; acute exacerbation of a chronic condition is likely to trigger the need for a difficult-to-predict amount of medical or nursing care.

A payments system such as the one described here would be based upon services that could be easily incorporated into the existing long-term-care-delivery system. The system would not reduce the current fragmentation of services across multiple programs, however. The recipient would still be faced with a bewildering array of different eligibility and copayment requirements for different types of services. An alternative arrangement would be to consolidate all long-term-care services (medical, nursing, and personal care) into a single benefit package with uniform eligibility requirements, but for the reasons cited here, the disability-payment mechanism may not be compatible with this more comprehensive approach.

Method of Payment

Benefits could be provided to recipients either as cash or as vouchers earmarked for any one among a specified set of long-term-care services. Conventional economic wisdom has favored cash over vouchers; cash transfers presumably maximize consumer sovereignty while minimizing market intervention. Thurow (1974) has argued, however, that this doctrine may not always be correct and that vouchers may be preferable under certain conditions such as when consumer sovereignty is limited. When some individuals are not competent to make certain decisions, society may use vouchers to induce these persons to make the "right" choice. Incompetence in this context is not restricted to mental deficiency but also could include ignorance and poor personal- or family-management ability.

Another condition favoring vouchers is the societal desire to equalize provision of a given service while still maintaining an unequal distribution of other goods and services. These societal preferences are often revealed through the political process. Thus, for example, society may wish to guarantee equal rights to medical care but not an equal distribution of income. Thurow (1974) argues that this equality can only be accomplished with vouchers or the in-kind distribution of medical care.

In order to resolve the issue of cash versus vouchers, two questions should be addressed. First, is there evidence for limited consumer sovereignty on the part of the disabled elderly? Second, is the equal distribution of long-term-care services part of our social-welfare function? A positive response to either question would suggest that a noncash program, hopefully one with the most attributes similar to cash (for example, vouchers), should be selected.

A more detailed description of all voucher and cash transfer systems is presented now in the following sections.

Vouchers. Under a voucher system, eligible recipients could purchase any of a specified set of long-term-care services. The range of covered services might in fact be quite broad, although limited to individuals deemed appropriate by program specifications. The primary advantage of this approach is that it would help ensure that recipients purchase long-term-care services rather than something else. Within these limits the individual consumer would still have control over the mix and quantity of services obtained, subject to the dollar constraint of the voucher.

Under a voucher system, quality assurance should be a part of program specifications. Minimal acceptable levels of quality could be assured through licensure or approval of providers. Vouchers then could be used only to obtain services from qualified providers. Federal housing allowance benefits, for example, are made only to residents of "adequate" dwellings, where adequacy is measured by building and safety codes and verified by inspection. However, standard setting and enforcement are apt to be extremely costly in any program, particularly when the number of providers is high. Regulating services provided by family members may be especially difficult. Program planners might explicitly assume minimum quality levels for family-provided care. The question of how to assure that minimum standards are observed by other nonprofessionals such as homemakers or personal-care attendants would still remain.

In-kind transfer programs are based on a concept of limited consumer sovereignty. Public policymakers assume that consumers may not always be competent to maximize their own utility and that societal preferences may be maximized by supplementing individual consumer judgments. Thus, the food stamp program, for example, assumes that some households may not be able to reach desired minimum nutritional levels and that this inefficiency can be offset by vouchers earmarked for food purchases.

However, vouchers may discourage efficient consumption in other ways. The recipients are less sensitive to price differences than they would be if they had to pay for the service themselves. With vouchers, savings accrued from thrifty shopping allow the individual to purchase more long-term-care services but not more of some other goods. As a result, the recipient with lower preferences for long-term care may overconsume services. Were he given cash, on the other hand, this consumer would, most likely, spend less on long-term care and more on other services. Of course to the extent that the consumer is able to meet all long-term care needs with his voucher, he will be able to reserve total income for other goods and services.

Copayments might be incorporated into a voucher system. Under this arrangement, a beneficiary would be required to pay some fraction of the face value of the vouchers before actually receiving them. A copayment system has the major advantage of being relatively antiinflationary. The consumer and/or his agent will be more sensitive to price and therefore more likely to use resources efficiently than under a pure voucher system. At the same time, however, uniform cost-sharing will fall disproportionately on the poor (Davis and Reynolds 1976). One alternative is to vary copayment rates with income or to set a ceiling on the total amount any one family would have to pay (possibly zero for the very poor and then raise the ceilings with income). Another approach would be to allow state Medicaid programs to "buy in" the copayments for the poor, as many of them have done under Medicare.

Several types of voucher systems for long-term care have already been discussed by Pollak (1974). One such system that is different from the one proposed here is an open-ended system in which the quantity of vouchers eligible individuals can receive is unlimited. On the one hand, copayments would be absolutely necessary to keep program costs within reasonable levels. This type of voucher system would not necessitate a complex client assessment to determine the level of benefits, and hence administrative costs would be minimized. On the other hand, whether such a program would be efficient in enabling those most at risk to purchase the services they need in order to remain in the community is unclear.

Cash Transfers. Under a cash-transfer program, benefits would be paid in cash to the beneficiary, who then would be responsible for purchasing all desired long-term-care services. He would be free both to shop for the best buy and to determine the actual mix of services. Savings accrued (from thrifty shopping, for example, or from services obtained gratis from family members) would not reduce benefit levels, but could be used to purchase other desired goods and services. The quantity of purchased services would be constrained only by the total size of the cash grant. Unlike the voucher system, cash grants would not require any licensing or certification of providers. Quality services would be provided only to the extent that consumers were willing to pay for them. By maximizing consumer sovereignty, cash transfers are generally assumed to result in more efficient resource use than under restricted grant programs.

The efficiency of cash transfers is predicated on the existence of both consumer sovereignty and competitive markets. However, consumer ignorance of what benefits could accrue from certain social and health care services and of what constitutes a fair price may make it difficult for the disabled elderly to shop for services. The physical and mental impairments of this population may raise information and research costs and may also leave them vulnerable to exploitation. In addition, the recipient may use some or all of his grant to purchase nonlong-term-care-related goods and services. Such goods might range from improvements in housing and nutrition to luxury items (the aged's version of welfare Cadillacs). Besides seriously jeopardizing political support for the program, this factor could have long-running social consequences as well. Externalities resulting from failure to utilize necessary services might include accelerated deterioration of health, increased hospital and nursing home admissions, and higher overall expenditures.

Finally, the assumption of a competitive long-term-care market may not be justified. To the extent that providers can induce demand for their services, utilization may be biased upward and toward more expensive forms of care.

A number of objections have been raised to a cash payment program. Pollak (1974) notes three fundamental deficiencies of such a program. First, in some areas demand may be too small to generate competition among providers and may not, therefore, reduce costs. Second, some individuals will not be capable of selecting a service package for themselves. Finally, political support may be weak for a program that permits neglect of some of the problems created by impairment, even if this neglect results from patient choice. Correia (1976) also faults a cash payment system by asserting it is "unworkable" for a number of reasons. First, the program is very difficult to administer and potentially very costly. Second, it encourages individuals to exaggerate their level of disability in order to receive higher payments.

The argument in favor of cash transfers, however, is supported by the evidence from abroad. Tracy (1974), whose findings are discussed in the following section, describes the nonwork-related disability payments in other industrialized countries. While most countries offer some form of cash assistance, no mention is made of a voucher system. Thurow's (1974) argument, in light of this fact, should be seriously considered: "While it is not axiomatically true that cash transfers always dominate restricted transfers, the general economic case for cash transfers is strong enough that the burden of proof should always lie on those who advocate restricted transfers."

Evidence from Abroad

As noted previously, disability payment programs are common abroad. Tracy reports the experience of forty-seven countries that provide constant attendance allowances to disabled persons who require full or part-time home care. This trend represents an effort, he asserts, "to contain the spiralling cost of providing long-term hospital or nursing home care by cash assistance designed to keep the beneficiary at home" (Tracy 1974, p. 32). Historically, benefits have been provided to disabled workers under workmen's compensation; more recently, however, programs have been instituted that have been directed toward coverage for persons with nonwork-related disabilities.

A disability allowance has been deemed necessary by many nations to fill the gaps left by the three other main programs that provide care to the disabled: workmen's compensation, home help services, and nursing homes. Many disabled individuals are not eligible for the benefits of workmen's compensation; some may need medical care not offered by home help agencies, and still others may shun the notion of entering a nursing home. Only three of the industrialized countries of the world do *not* offer such an allowance: the United States, Canada, and West Germany. In most other nations the disability allowance is paid as a supplement to the invalidity component of a social insurance program.

Eligibility is usually granted to individuals who have lost two-thirds of their working capacity and who have contributed from their salary to Social Security. Usually, to receive a supplement, the person must require help with the activities of daily living for at least twelve hours a day. In some countries, however, lesser degrees of disability are also covered. Determination of the level of disability is usually carried out by the individual's personal physician. Most countries employ a means test, under which a person receives an allowance only if his income falls below a determined level; certain countries include the family's income as well.

Benefits are usually computed as a percentage of the recipient's invalidity pension; some countries, however, determine payment levels according to the worker's average earnings. Seven countries (Australia Czechoslovakia, Finland, Poland, Romania, South Africa, United Kingdom) provide a flat-rate, fixed allowance. Funds to pay for constant attendance allowances come from the payroll deductions that support normal invalidity pensions.

Tracy describes three more recent programs that are more germane to the proposed disability allowance model. In 1973, Australia initiated a flat-rate benefit of $2.00 Australian ($3.00 American) a day, paid to persons caring for an elderly relative at home. France established a means-tested program in 1971 that provides a sum to help cover home care for nonelderly handicapped individuals. In 1970, the United Kingdom began to provide a constant attendance supplement for individuals with severe, nonwork-related handicaps.

Evaluation

In order to evaluate the potential advantages and disadvantages of this option, it is necessary to specify the parameters in more detail, since as discussed in the previous section, a great variety of alternative methods exist of establishing a disability allowance program, and the ramifications of several of these programs are widely disparate. It will be assumed in what follows that the disability allowance will be in the form of vouchers and that these vouchers will be used to pay for social support services including such services as assistance with personal care, homemaking chores, and transportation services, but the allowance will not include payment for medical, skilled nursing, or other therapeutic services.[3] No means test will be required for eligibility, but there will be a copayment—that is, the vouchers will be purchased by the recipient. This copayment may be covered in part by Medicaid or may vary with income level, so that low income individuals will not be prevented from using the program.

Under the proposed model, vouchers will be distributed by local agencies that will be responsible also for assessing the individual's functional status in a number of areas, including physical functioning, intellectual functioning, personal adjustment, physical health/medical status, and social contact. The specification of what agency or agencies would be appropriate is beyond the scope of this book. An overall judgment regarding each individual's functional level would be made by the person carrying out the assessment. For example, if one used the scheme employed in the Cleveland GAO study (Comptroller General of the United States 1977), which is based on the assessment instrument (developed by the Older Americans Resources and Services Project (OARS) at Duke University, seven levels of impairment would result: unimpaired, slightly impaired, mildly impaired, moderately impaired, generally impaired, greatly impaired, and extremely impaired. Seven different payment levels could be associated with each of these disability or impairment levels (Comptroller General of the United States 1977). The actual dollar value of vouchers distributed would depend not only on disability level but also upon living arrangements—individuals living alone would receive a higher benefit voucher payment than those at the same disability level who reside with their spouse or other family member. Benefit voucher payments would also be made to individuals who choose to live in a foster or personal care home or other type of domicilary care facility. The benefit structure—that is, the amount of vouchers distributed—would be constructed in such a manner as to provide incentives to the individual to select the most cost-effective option. Thus, at low-impairment levels, few or no benefit vouchers would be distributed to individuals choosing the domicilary-care option, while at higher levels of impairment, the benefits paid to individuals choosing the domiciliary care option would be more nearly equal to those provided to individuals who choose to remain in the community.

In order to avoid abuse, providers would be required to register with the assessment agency. Only registered providers would be permitted to obtain cash for vouchers received. The provider could be an agency but might also be an individual. No licensing of providers would be required.

Framework of the Evaluation

The following analysis primarily relates to the specific option proposed in the last section; where appropriate, however, mention is made of other variations in possible disability allowance programs. For example, even though a voucher system was proposed, the effects of a cash transfer system are also briefly analyzed.

Coverage. The program is likely to result in the coverage of more persons and an expansion of services. Presently, elderly individuals are provided long-term care under service programs such as Medicare. With the proposed model, elderly people would receive a disability allowance with which they could purchase services for themselves. General consensus is that existing programs do not offer sufficient coverage to help individuals to avoid unnecessary institutionalization. Probably the disability allowance would extend benefits to a wider range of consumers, from those with few personal care needs to the severely disabled.

An expansion of services would result from the new relationship between consumer and provider that would emerge under this program. Instead of being constrained by the restrictions on what third party payors will reimburse, providers would be able to offer a wide range of alternative services. In addition, the elderly person possibly could contract with a friend, relative, or neighbor for services, expanding even further the potential pool of service providers.

Funding of Program. A substantial amount of the funds needed to support a disability allowance could come from the reallocation of resources from existing programs. Since individuals would receive vouchers to purchase services, funds for existing service-providing programs such as Title XX could be reduced. In addition, administrative costs will be lower under a disability allowance program, as much of the paperwork, bill paying, and monitoring will be obviated. Savings achieved in this fashion could be applied to an increase in disability payments and/or in the number of individuals covered.

As noted before, however, many elderly persons are needlessly institutionalized because of their unmet need for assistance in the home. In order to have a significant effect on this problem, the disability allowance would have to be large enough to enable the individual to purchase a sufficient amount of home care services to remain at home. Since it is generally agreed that existing programs are inadequate, additional funds would need to be allocated to make the program truly effective. This need will become still more likely if coverage is expanded to new groups of less severely disabled elderly.

In summary, while reallocation of funds will cover some of the expense of the program, additional appropriations would undoubtedly be necessary.

Effect on Consumers. The most positive aspect of this approach would be its effect on consumers. Impaired individuals would have much greater freedom of choice with respect to choosing community living arrangements instead of institutional ones and choosing particular providers. Recipients of the allowance would be able to control to some extent the quality of the service they receive by "taking their business elsewhere" if they are unsatisfied. If consumers were allowed to apply the allowance towards institutional care, a similar advantage would result. Nursing homes with low standards of care and poor reputations could be deserted by consumers with greater purchasing power.

Access to help would be increased for the very old and severely disabled. Their disability allowance would, on the average, be higher, presuming that a sliding scale based on disability level is used to determine the level of benefits. The poor would gain greater access to basic services and would thus be able to remain home longer. While the effect would be less dramatic on the nonpoor, a disability allowance would permit them to purchase nonessential but desirable services such as companionship or respite care.

Potential for Program Abuse. The possibilities for abuse are two-fold: (1) abuse by those receiving the allowance and (2) by those caring for recipients. Since the central element of this program is *case management* by the consumer, for constraints to be put on the way the individual uses the allowance is not desirable. If, however, the program is used for nonessential luxury items, a political backlash might develop that could jeopardize the program. This problem, however, exists much more strongly in a cash system. With the proposed voucher, consumer choice will be circumscribed. A copayment acts as additional encouragement to a savings-conscious mentality among consumers.

Abuse by family and providers is a more serious issue. The question of *free consumer choice* becomes less relevant if the individual is so severely physically, or more important, mentally impaired that rational decision making is impossible. Such a person could be easily taken advantage of, unless some mechanism existed to monitor the most severely disabled. An important recommendation is that a consumer-advocacy element be included in the program to fulfill this function. The agency that evaluates the client, for example, could determine the need for an advocate and could provide one if necessary.

Another negative aspect of the proposed program is that it does not deal with the problem associated with achieving proper coordination of care for an impaired person in need of a complex range of services. While a central aspect of a disability payment program is the placement of the case management function in the hands of the consumer, many consumers may not know how and where to obtain services. Possibly, consumers who have difficulty arranging the provision of services for themselves can be identified and provided assistance in doing so.

Family Involvement. As has been noted at various points throughout this chapter, one of the questions most difficult to resolve is the effect that this option may have on the support provided to the individual by the family. The central dilemma is as follows. Disabled individuals who have no family are in greater need of formal support in order to remain in the home, which could indicate that they should receive a higher disability allowance. However, this aspect could have the perverse effect of encouraging families to push an elder member into a more independent living status to receive a larger payment. Since lower-class families more often take in elderly relatives, it is precisely these people who might receive less of an allowance and, hence, be more disinclined to have an elderly relation live with them.

A possible solution is to provide an elderly person living with relatives an allowance smaller than for a similar person living alone but to make available respite care as a free service in each community. This service would reduce the stress of the care-giving family and also would take into account the needs of the isolated individual. A second possibility would be to reduce or eliminate the copayment for the person living alone. Before the enactment of disability allowance, this issue must be carefully evaluated in the light of any empirical findings that exist. Any reduction in the amount of care provided by families to the severely disabled is highly undesirable and should be carefully avoided.

Effect on Providers. As stated previously, individuals receiving a disability allowance would have greater freedom to choose among particular providers. Assuming the disability payment levels were high enough,[4] the increased demand for services would generate an increasing supply of personal and other home care services, as well as sheltered living arrangements. This demand would encourage competition among providers. This increased competition, coupled with the change in focus from a single purchaser (the government) to multiple purchasers (consumers), likely would lead to improvements in the quality of services.

In the case of home care services, efficiency in delivery might improve as older persons shop around to find the most competitively priced alternatives. Home care agencies would, if the option permits, also have to compete against the informal personal care services that the elderly could purchase. In general, competition would be created in the market, and more efficient delivery could result.

Changes in the mix of services and in the allocation of public dollars probably would result from this option. The proposed allowance would pay for nonmedical services, and coverage would be extended to individuals previously unable to purchase such services who thus could now do so. An increase in the utilization would in turn increase the availability of home care services, while no such increase in medical services would result. Public funds would very likely be shifted from institutional to noninstitutional services, since this program should result in keeping some individuals out of institutions.

An increase in flexibility of the use of services also may result from a disability allowance program. At present, certain governmental restrictions are imposed on the services that can be provided to an elderly person. For example, Medicare will not pay for home-delivered meals or homemaker services but will pay for part-time skilled nursing care. The consumers, however, will be given an allowance to spend as they wish; providers can respond by offering new and alternative services. Thus, the patients are likely to receive services more closely tailored to their needs and not merely what is made available by a fiscal intermediary such as Medicare.

Distribution of Costs. Initially, a decrease in costs borne by relatives may be expected. In families that care for an elderly person, the allowance could be applied to basic services that would allow a member to work or to leave the home for some other reason. If the program achieves its aims, however, it will enable impaired elderly persons to remain in the community for a longer time. Hopefully, the disability allowance will supplement the help available from family and friends, thus relieving some of the burden on these informal providers, and thereby reducing the likelihood that the impaired person would be institutionalized. The total costs actually borne by relatives may increase rather than decrease, since the individual will stay with his or her family for a longer period of time.

If the disability allowance program is successful, it will lead to a decrease in institutionalization, and a decrease in costs borne by the federal and state governments would offset all, or at least part, of the additional expenditures needed to make the disability payments. Determination of how savings would be distributed between the federal government and the states must remain unresolved until the sources of funding for the program are decided upon.

Administrative costs will be lower for a disability allowance program as compared with most other options, in which a large proportion of long-term-care funds are spent on case management and related activities that revolve around making up a care plan for clients. With a disability allowance this spending would be unnecessary in all but the severest cases. The elderly recipients themselves will be their own case managers. Further savings will result from the elimination of paperwork that exists in a fee-for service-payment system. At present, the government must evaluate and pay a bill for each service a client receives; under a disability allowance program, the client would pay for each service himself. A voucher system will reduce the expense of paperwork less than a cash system, as the vouchers will have to be processed. Savings may be offset as well by the monitoring or advocacy system that would be developed for the severely mentally or physically impaired.

Organizational Issues. As emphasized at different points throughout this discussion, much of the control would be lodged with the consumer. The only authority allocated to the government would be the establishment of the levels of payment and the eligibility requirements. Once these factors are determined, almost total control over service mix and utilization would be placed in the hands of the consumer.

Providers, however, would also gain new freedom to experiment with alternative services. At present, they are somewhat constrained by the limitations on what is reimbursable by third party payors. Under this program, the market is restored to some extent, enabling providers to compete with one another to improve and expand their services and to engage in creative service planning to attract new customers. Thus, the authority of the government bureaucracy and of third party payors is expected to diminish.

Political and Economic Feasibility. Under close analysis, the arguments for or against disability allowance programs clearly are rooted in more serious political and philosophical beliefs. The essential question, also posed by Thurow (1974), is this: Does society want to encourage the individual to exercise free choice even if this means possible abuse? Or is a paternalistic view more tenable, which in this case would indicate that there are certain things individuals *should* have, whether they necessarily want them or not? Although these questions are not answered here, all parties involved in the planning of such an option must be aware of them.

A second political issue, which has been touched on before, revolves around potential abuse of the program by both providers and consumers.

Certainly, potential for abuse is greater in this program than in the organizational reforms presented later. If widespread misuse of the allowance took place, a political reaction against this program might take place, which could also extend to other long-term-care programs. This outcome is particularly undesirable in the light of the present Proposition 13, cost-cutting mentality. The agency administrating these allowances hopefully can serve as a force to prevent the occurrence of widespread abuse.

Third, the effect of this option on the delicate balance between formal and informal supports must be carefully evaluated. If the size of the allowance is based on family status, the undesired effect of encouraging families to abandon the elderly person could result. This effect would increase the cost of the program tremendously. Some mechanism must be developed to encourage families to continue to support an elderly relative, while providing the greater amount of care that an isolated, impaired individual needs. Further research is needed to resolve this question.

Another issue of major importance is that of the severely disabled, isolated elderly. In order for a disability allowance to be economically feasible, payments would have to be substantially lower than the real cost of care. Presumably, since 60-80 percent of the costs are being borne by relatives, the allowance will not cover 100 percent of the expense—only expense not provided by the family. Otherwise, the cost of the program would be prohibitively high and might result in the substitution of formal for informal supports. If, however, the proposed model implies the abandonment of all other programs, and their replacement with a disability allowance (possibly as low as $200-$300 per month), then it would seem that the severely impaired elderly could run a greater risk of institutionalization than under any of the other proposed options. This issue needs to be clarified and resolved in order to insure the viability of a disability allowance program.

One final caveat remains to be mentioned here. Disability payments, by shifting some of the locus of control from the third party payor to the consumer, would undoubtedly have important secondary effects on the relationship among providers as well as that between consumers and providers. One major likely effect that stands out is an undesirable one: a further fragmentation of health, social, and other home support services is likely to arise because of the fragmentary nature of the payment system—(that is, the fact that it will pay for only unskilled services). It is true that for many disabled individuals, the most important services lacking are the personal care, homemaker, and chore services. Nonetheless, many of these individuals have a significant need for medical care services that would be financed separately under the proposed system. Within this model, coordinating the medical and nonmedical services would seem to be difficult without an intricate case management approach. Such an approach would not be consistent in principle with the disability payment system.

Notes

1. Workmen's Compensation is a third program providing benefits to the disabled. It is administered by state governments and provides insurance against industrial accidents and occupational diseases. Because of the special purpose of this program it is not discussed in this analysis.

2. Medicare Part A provides a maximum of one hundred home-health units, following a minimum three-day hospitalization. The beneficiary care extends home-health service under Part B for an additional one hundred units, but he must also pay the 20-percent coinsurance. Visits by all providers (registered nurse, home-health aid, physical therapists, and so on) are counted towards this ceiling.

3. Although arguments in favor of the particular model discussed here were presented in the previous section, the authors feel that other alternatives (one being a cash program) could also provide certain advantages.

4. The price level is not the only issue. The density of potential users will also be important in determining the degree to which increases in supply are stimulated.

References

Callahan, Jr., James J., Diamond, Lawrence D., Giele, Janet Z., and Morris, Robert. 1980. "Responsibility of Families for their Severely Disabled Elders." University Health Policy Consortium, Brandeis University. In *Health Care Financing Review* 1 (3):29-48.

Chiswick, B.R. 1976. "The Demand for Nursing Home Care: An Analysis of the Substitution Between Institutional and Noninstitutional Care." *The Journal of Human Resources* 11 (Summer):295-316.

Comptroller General of the United States, 1977. *The Well-Being of Older People in Cleveland, Ohio.* GAO Report to the Congress, April 19.

Correia, E. 1976. "National Health Insurance, Welfare Reform, and the Disabled: Issues in Program Reform." Paper prepared for Office of the Assistant Secretary for Planning and Evaluation, U.S. Department of Health, Education, and Welfare, Washington, D.C., August.

Davis, J.W. and Gibbon, M.J. 1971. "An Areawide Examination of Nursing Home Use, Misuse and Nonuse." *American Journal of Public Health* 61 (June):1146-1155.

Davis, K., and Reynolds, R. 1976. "The Impact of Medicare and Medicaid on Access to Medical Care." In *The Role of Health Insurance in the Health Services Sector,* ed. Richard Rosett, pp. 391-425. New York: National Bureau of Economic Research.

Frohlich P. 1971. "Who are the Disabled in Institutions?" *Social Security Bulletin* 34 (October):3-10.

Grossman, M.J. 1972. *The Demand for Health: A Theoretical and Empirical Analysis.* New York: Columbia University Press.

Nash, D.T. 1966. "Home Care for the Chronically Institutionalized." *Geriatrics* 21 (February):215-220.

Pettigrew, A., and Kinloch, D. 1971. Background Information on Proposed Rules and Regulations for Long-Term Care Facilities. Unpublished paper for Massachusetts Department of Public Health, January 12.

National Center for Health Statistics. 1979. "The National Nursing Home Survey: 1977 Summary for the United States." *Vital and Health Statistics* Series 13, Number 43. Data from the National Health Survey, U.S. Department of Health, Education, and Welfare, July.

Pollak, W. 1974. *Federal Long-Term Care Strategy: Options and Analysis.* Washington, D.C.: Urban Institute, February 25.

Sussman, M. 1979. "Social and Economic Supports and Family Environments for the Elderly." Final Report to Administration on Aging, AOA Grant #90-A316(03) Winston-Salem, N.C.: Wake Forest University and Bowman Grey School of Medicine.

Thurow, L.C. 1974. "Cash versus In-Kind Transfers." *American Economic Review.* 64 (May):190-195.

Tracy, M. 1974. "Constant Attendance Allowance for Non-Work Related Disability." *Social Security Bulletin* 37 (November):32-37.

Wilder, C.S. 1977. "Limitation of Activity Due to Chronic Conditions, United States, 1974." *Vital and Health Statistics* Series 10, Data from the National Health Survey No. 111. Washington, D.C.: National Center for Health Statistics, U.S. Department of Health, Education, and Welfare, June.

Williams, Franklin T., et al. 1973. "Appropriate Placement of the Chronically Ill and Aged." *Journal of the American Medical Association* 226 (December 10):1332-1335.

Part III
Options for Organizing
Long-Term Care

The options considered for organizing the delivery of long-term-care services are the case management concept, the single agency model, and the social/health maintenance organization (S/HMO). In a period of fiscal constraint, organizational structural change may be feasible as it adopts a new approach to an already existing network.

Dennis Beatrice in chapter 6 presents a detailed analysis of the case management concept and shows how case management might be the most immediate device available for improving the life of persons with long-term-care needs. Beatrice discusses the system structure into which case management would be inserted. He defines and discusses "identifiable case management functions ranging from data collection, to assessment, to follow-up." Beatrice sees the variables of authority, location, and assessment style as issues to be resolved prior to the establishment of any case management system. A point reinforced over and over again by Beatrice is his belief that local environments are critical in shaping the case management process. A prototypical model is offered and discussed, and the chapter concludes with the recommendation for an incremental approach. While Beatrice points out that a redesigned case management system can be viewed as a reform option, the specifics of case management described can be integrated into other reform proposals.

James Callahan, in his discussion of a single agency model in chapter 7, also recommends incrementalism. Callahan reviews a number of single agency efforts of some other demonstrations. Drawing upon systems concepts presented in more detail in chapter 9, he identifies compatible and incompatible functions and suggests a model that builds on mutually reinforcing functions. Local agencies that might serve as a single agency are identified and a detailed analysis of the Area on Aging is presented. Callahan calls for the separation of financing, planning, and advocacy from service delivery.

Larry Diamond and David Berman in chapter 8 present the concept of a new entity—the (S/HMO)—as a way of bridging the financing and delivery of long-term-care services. They call for a prepaid, capitated organization that offers a full range of medical and social services to an enrolled population over age sixty-five. Having to operate within a fixed per capita budget is presented as a means to shift care from high-cost institutional services to lower-cost, ambulatory community- and personal-care services. While the

S/HMO is presented as an exciting innovation, the authors candidly review the problems of enrollment, risk sharing, cost cutting, and quality of care. The need for the federal government to be more creative in helping such organizations get off the ground is noted.

Case Management, a Single Agency, and a Social/Health Maintenance Organization are three particular ways of organizing long-term-care functions. Certainly other arrangements are possible. In chapter 9, Callahan takes a systems approach to the long-term-care field. He identifies the functions, components, levels, and key agencies in this sector. These are the building blocks for different forms of long-term-care networks and/or organization. Callahan's chapter is useful both for its completeness and specificity.

6

Case Management: A Policy Option for Long-Term Care

Dennis F. Beatrice

Service integration and *coordination* have become the modern equivalents of the philosopher's stone, through which social service planners seek to turn the "lead" of disconnected-service programs into the "gold" of organized, consistent services that actually address client need and do so without waste. This search for coordination has grown over time, in response to issues such as the increase in services and coverage; the expansion of narrow, categorical programs with their own authorizations, regulations, and operational styles; the growth in the pool of individuals seeking services; the greater recognition of need; and the emergence of social service professionals who see and react to human need and attempt to affect the service system to meet the needs observed.

Long-term-care services have not been immune from the effort to organize and coordinate. Since a patchwork maze of programs and service types exists to address the long-term-care requirements of people with special and diverse needs, the cry for coordination has often arisen. *Case management* is often posited as the vehicle by which long-term-care services are to be integrated and coordinated.

Case management is seen as a way to address a series of problems perceived in the way long-term-care services are organized and delivered. These difficulties include:

Fragmentation of services and programs,

Service gaps,

Duplication,

Programs' working at cross-purposes,

A lack of comprehensiveness in service arrangement and delivery,

The fact that long-term-care clients evidence multiple needs that can be addressed only by a coordinated service approach.

Case management attempts to treat these problems by:

Integrating and individualizing long-term-care services;

Helping clients gain access to a continuum of services;

Assuring that services given are appropriate for the problem of a particular client;

Facilitating the development of a broader array of noninstitutional services. Case management thus works to lessen maldistribution of resources within the system and to increase total dollar flow to the sector in the form of new services;

Following clients to guarantee continued appropriateness of service;

Assuring that services are provided in a coordinated way to meet multiple and diverse client needs.

This chapter discusses in detail the range of possible case management models and the permutations of possible goals and functions. However, it is possible to suggest basic characteristics of a case management system that will:

Be comprised of a network of case-managing entities, somehow arrayed, that receive referrals of individuals in need of long-term-care services;

Conduct broad initial-need assessment;

Recommend appropriate services in the context of a service plan that is time limited and that stresses consideration of all service options;

Connect clients to services and work to develop "service packages" that incorporate the services needed by individual clients;

Reexamine clients' progress periodically and revise the plan to reflect changes in service need or environmental-support factors.

It is important to note that case management is the long-term-care policy option being discussed here. Case management of some sort will probably be an ingredient in any system change undertaken, but for the purposes of the discussion of this option, case management is the only change being implemented. The purpose of this analysis is to consider the implications of changing the current long-term-care-service system only by adding a broad case-management component to it. A strategy of coordination must be understood as a reform in its own terms. It follows from a belief that services are "better" when they are coordinated and that fragmentation within a system is less desirable than comprehensiveness.

The purpose of proposing a case management system is to change the way in which the long-term-care-service system affects clients. Currently, the client or a helper must be sufficiently sophisticated and facile to "use" the system to his or her advantage. If the client does not interact with the system effectively, it affects him or her in an ill-defined and variable manner. Case management postulates an environment in which a case management structure takes the responsibility for making the system work for the client in a consistent and coherent manner. It relieves at least some of the burden from the individual client attempting to grapple with a serpentine service system.

Case management also aims to optimize the level of service that can be provided with a given level of funding by increasing the efficiency and effectiveness of service delivery. As funding of new programs begins to slow down and as increasing restrictions are placed on the funding of existing programs, maximizing benefits derived from existing resources will become increasingly important. A commitment to case management is a policy to maximize resources through the integration and individualization of benefits available from existing programs. Unique mixes of long-term care are needed to maximize the effectiveness of public funds, and case management is predicated on building the service system from the level of unique individual need.

Another result of a broader commitment to case management is the potential for an overall improvement in the "image of competence" held by the public for administrators of long-term-care services. All elderly individuals can feel that someone is there to whom they can turn for assistance, who can rationalize the maze of service programs and types. The public as a whole can see case management as a consumer-oriented entity, committed to "rescuing" persons from the maw of public programs and bureaucracy. The clients aided by case management will see it as a public program uniquely available for their benefit.

The chapter examines:

System structure: Shows how the features of a particular long-term-care-service environment should and will affect the way case management is implemented;

Case management functions: Examines the broad range of potential case management functions;

Case management-program-design issues: Discusses a series of questions and issues that must be addressed in the implementation of any case-management system;

Constructing a case management model: Environmental Map and Service System—discusses how the current long-term-care system is arrayed, how case management will alter the system, and how case management will function within the new arrangements it facilitates;

A prototypical case management model: Makes assumptions about the infinite permutations of possible goals, functions, and design issues to yield a model case management system for analysis;

Effects and implications of case management: Discusses relative organizational and administrative issues, political and economic feasibility, cost implications, and effects on consumers, providers, and coverage of services.

The chapter discusses the structure and implications of case management, with a special focus on explaining how case management may be used to bridge the gap between the long-term-care-service benefits available and the ones that eligible recipients desire to obtain. It attempts to delineate the parameters of how a case management structure can act on the present system to improve matching, assessment, access, quality, and cost-effectiveness.

Case Management Variations

One may envision many possible case management variations. A fine-tuned assessment of the particular environment (state or substate region) into which case management is to be introduced would generate reasons to structure case management differently. Case management must respond to the particular characteristics and needs of the particular system within which it is to integrate and coordinate.

Case management is therefore neither inherently nor definitively defined. It derives its definition in large part from the nature and needs of a system whose component parts it will be coordinating and integrating. We will suggest that case management has some relatively immutable features and characteristics but that it must be a creature of its environment, tuned to the specific characteristics and needs of its host system, if it is to be effective. The manifestations of case management are broad, as evidenced by the range of case management demonstrations functioning in Connecticut, New York, Wisconsin, Washington, and Massachusetts. Additional variations on the basic theme could emerge in different settings to answer different needs or perform different functions.

Case management will vary along three dimensions.

System structure: The features of a particular system should and will affect the way case management is implemented. States have different needs relative to their long-term-care systems. Case management will and/or should adjust itself to those differences, if not out of rationality than from an understanding that a square peg in a round hole neither fits nor works well.

Case management functions: Case management can perform a broad range of functions. Decisions as to which functions will be performed, which will be emphasized, and which will be excluded are important. The mix of functions chosen will thus affect case management organization and activity.

Case management-program-design issues: A series of questions and issues must be addressed by any case management system. The issues relate to the authority, assessment style, and location (within the system) of the case management structure being contemplated.

The development of case management can be considered as a four-step process. First, the structure of the system into which it will become embedded must be understood. This understanding is the basis for structuring a useful and productive case management role. Second, partially in response to the first analysis about system structure, case management functions must be identified. Preferably, the functions to be performed will parallel the needs observed in the system and fit comfortably with the characteristics and nature of that system. Third, the questions of organization and spillover effects must be answered. Again, these answers should reference the preceding analyses; it will only be possible to answer intelligently the questions posed by case management if the system's needs, characteristics, and nature are understood and if, in response to these, case management functions are delineated. With an understanding of what case management is to do in a given milieu, it will be possible to answer the questions that are endemic to case management. Finally, the case management system, cognizant of system needs, secure in its functions, and adequately arrayed after having addressed its fundamental questions, will be implemented as a coordinating/integrating/individualizing device.

Let us turn now to a review of the three dimensions that affect case management: system structure, functions, and program-design issues. The most appropriate model for case management flows from the choices made in these three areas. No one program model suits all states or communities. The case management functions must serve different needs, in different circumstances, at different times. The core of a commitment to case management as an option for long-term-care-service-delivery improvement is a decision to attempt to lessen institutionalization. The method to be pursued is to maximize the use of noninstitutional services through the use of a client-oriented coordinating/integrating/individualizing mechanism. The most appropriate way to effectuate the decision to pursue these goals is the issue addressed in the remainder of this chapter.

System Structure

The first consideration necessary when case management is being contemplated is the status of the system with which it will interface. Characteristics of that system must affect the nature of the case management structure. Case management will function differently depending on its environment. Some items to consider within the environment are:

Capacity: No gains accrue from coordinating incompetent or irrelevant services. The focus of case management will depend on the infrastructure of services that exists to manage. The emphasis will be shifted among the goals of facilitating or directing service development, integrating existing services, or "running interference" through a maze of complex services with conflicting and complex entry rules depending on the availability of existing services. However arrayed, case management is predicated on the notion of utilizing existing services in a more productive way. Therefore, the existing service capacity must, by its absence or presence, affect case management.

Complexity: Long-term-care systems vary in their complexity at a minimum in terms of: size, number of providers involved, at-risk population size, assessment technology, complexity of intergovernmental relations, complexity of interagency relationships within governmental levels, extent of private/proprietary sectors, activity level of consumer-advocacy groups, and authority relationships between agencies and actors.

The structural and functional characteristics of case management must consider this complexity. Obviously, case management will neither look nor function the same in environments of different complexity. A case management structure must be formulated so as to deal with diversity and complexity. The greater the systemic complexity faced, the greater must be the reach of the case management system to accommodate it.

Strength of the current service coordination and distribution network: Different systems coordinate and distribute their benefits with varying degrees of efficiency. The more effective the existing distribution/coordination system of long-term-care services, the less intense the need for case management. The more diffused and weak the distribution system and the less coherent the existing coordinating mechanisms, the more intense is the need for case management. If a system allocates resources efficiently under conditions of scarcity, case management is less essential. If resources are not distributed effectively, targeted properly, and allocated rationally and equitably, case management is needed more and should have a firmer grasp of its task—if one assumes that need (for allocation precision) translates into an opportunity to perform that allocation function. At any rate, the status of the existing distribution/allocation/coordination functions should affect how case management is structured, how openly it is received, and how badly it is needed.

Scope: Variations in the size of the long-term-care-service system will influence the form case management can adopt. The resources and effort necessary to process 300 admissions per month are different from those necessary to process 3,000 per month. As the number of intakes and interactions increases, the type of staffing required and the nature of the interactions must vary. The input of resources that can be made available is related to the number of claimants on those resources. The intensity of input that can reasonably be invested in each client is limited—resource limitations and administrative capacity will set the parameters. Therefore, the scope of the client population will affect case management structure. The depth of the interaction and the intensity of the case managment effort will be in inverse proportion to the number of individuals to be processed through the system—as client load (scope) increases, the intensity and depth of the intervention will decline. Fewer people can be served more intensely; more can be served less intensely.

Service gaps: As with capacity, the gaps that exist in the long-term-care, noninstitutional-service system will affect case management. Essential services are needed in a noninstitutionally oriented system. The type of services available will affect case management as will the extent (capacity) of the service network. Mental health planners have identified an essential range of services necessary to deinstitutionalization efforts. Long-term care requires an array of services if institutionalization is to be delayed or avoided. Case management will be differentially effective as this essential service array is or is not available. Coordination/integration/allocation/individualization are all circumscribed by the types of services available. Therefore, case management depends for its effectiveness and structure partially on the array of services on which it can draw.

Duplication: Case management bears a different burden if the delivery system is duplicative than if it is relatively well integrated. In an environment of duplication, case management must rationalize and routinize service flow. In an environment of scarcity, where insufficient rather than duplicative resources are the rule, case management must ration and target. The role of case management is quite different under different conditions of duplication in service.

Fragmentation: Long-term-care systems are more-or-less fragmented. Greater fragmentation increases the need for case management. If a service system is integrated, case management is superfluous. The problem can be viewed on a continuum—as fragmentation increases, the role of case management becomes clearer; as integration increases, the salience of case management is lessened.

Summary: Case management cannot be discussed without reference to particular long-term-care-service environments. Systemic features such as those discussed previously, affect the form and substance of case management. Case management as a generic function, understood to be an effort at coordination/integration/allocation/individualization within conditions of scarcity, can be advocated as an approach to long-term-care-service delivery and rationalization. However, it should be understood that the case management function must be tooled to fit its environment. Therefore, an assessment of the particular service system within which case management will function must precede and underlie the implementation of a case management program.

Case Management Functions

Case management can perform a broad range of functions in different systems. The most appropriate functions will flow from the features of the particular system, as discussed previously. The functions are not immutable; they are a response to the needs perceived in various environments. What is needed, and what case management should do, depends on what exists. Case management should fit its environment.

Depending on the characteristics of the particular long-term-care-service system and the needs evidenced and opportunities presented by that system, case management can serve the functions discussed in the following sections.

Data Collection

At a minimum, case management can document service gaps through data collection on its clients. A case management system, with no further role or authority, can help isolate why an institutional orientation exists in a given system. A case management structure can observe, on a case-by-case basis, if institutionalization occurs because noninstitutional-service capacity is limited, if gaps in essential types of service exist, or if family interactions and supports (or lack of supports) contribute significantly to institutionalization that, functionally speaking in terms of the individual, is inappropriate. The documentation of such realities can help long-term-care planners understand what is needed to increase the viability of the noninstitutional-service system. With this understanding comes the ability to present a more persuasive case to policymakers about specific needs within the noninstitutional service system.

Planning

Case management, as implied in the last section on its role of data collector, can be a planning tool, isolating areas of system balkiness, service gaps, lack of capacity, and other problems and developing possible responses to those dilemmas. The integration of a case management planning function (as opposed to a data collection or recording function) with other health planning entities would be a difficult task. Also, planners and service coordinators/integrators/individualizers are likely to have different skills. The latter function requires a sensitivity to need with a strong organizational and bureaucratic sense. The planner needs these characteristics too, but one can assert that the task of the planner is usually somewhat more removed from client contact and interaction and direct systemic manipulation. Case management will interface with the service planning process.

Public Educator

Case management can serve to educate at-risk individuals and their families about noninstitutional support services that could avert institutionalization. One can assert that some institutionalization is the result of insufficient information, that if individuals were apprised of available home support services, they would utilize them rather than seek institutional care. Irrespective of any further authority, a case manager can present this information and bolster the sense that home maintenance is a viable alternative, with proper support. The case manager then slips into his role of coordinator/integrator/allocator to devise a mix of support services that does make home maintenance viable and attractive. The "power to persuade" is an informal route that can be important in case management.

Resource to other Actors in the System

As the case management structure can educate the consumer, so it can educate suppliers of long-term-care services. Government agencies charged with long-term-care-service delivery (hospital-discharge planners, community-organization personnel, advocacy groups, and elderly-service groups) can all be served by the expertise of the case manager. This expertise is most likely to take the form of "system-manipulation specialization." The case management structure will, through its constant utilization of the component parts of the long-term-care system, become expert in the use of that system. This holistic view and understanding is likely to be greater than that of other participants in the service-referral/delivery process, since the others have a more localized mandate. The case manager's stress on system understanding and manipulation will establish him as someone to turn to for guidance.

Resource Locator

Educating the public and serving as a resource to related professionals can be part of the case management role. Flowing from these roles is a role as long-term-care-service locator. The case management system will adapt to traversing the maze of service options. Information about options will, in time, be obtainable most easily through the case manager. This situation will make the case management structure the obvious place for an individual or other actors in the system to which to turn for guidance in tapping available resources. Accessibility to services is enhanced by the presence of an identifiable, competent service facilitator. Case management can increase the chances that an individual who "stumbles" across an entry point to noninstitutional long-term-care services will receive a group of services. Disjointedness and randomness should be lessened. The service emphasis an individual receives should not be dictated by chance. Case management can increase access to a wider range of services and not hamstring an individual with one type of service that may or may not be most appropriate and sufficient.

"Triage Officer"

The case manager can do far more than collect data, educate the public, be a resource center, and locate and tap service resources. Case management can control entry to the long-term-care system. Case management can improve consumer information and choice by substituting for the informed consumer usually lacking information relative to long-term-care services. By supplying information, advice, or even making authoritative decisions, the case management function can comprise the rational, informed "purchaser" of service imputed into an operating market. Case management power functions along a continuum in this regard. The case manager can recommend or enforce, control, or monitor. Obviously, as we move toward enforcement and control, the ability to authoritatively allocate resources is increased. "Triage" is used consciously as a concept—under conditions of scarcity, a case management system hopefully can improve the flow of services, either toward persons most at risk of institutionalization or toward those who are in need of service resources but at a less intense and immediate level. "Targeting" services can be a crucial case management function—one that is more important if resources are limited or simply inadequate.

Assessment

A likely and probably unavoidable case management function is client assessment. The assessment process will direct the flow of individuals—

indicating which clients need institutionalization to deal with a physical or mental condition, which clients can be maintained in the community, what supports are needed, and which clients are institutionalized because of lack of noninstitutional-service resources. The assessment will also indicate the role of family or peer support; a key question in assessing the viability of community maintenance will be the availability and attitudes of this support structure. The case manager will help direct individuals toward noninstitutional services and may enforce level-of-care decisions. The reality will fall between persuasion and benefit denial; an individual will not be denied institutional service if noninstitutional service is inadequate, inappropriate, or if family supports are lacking. Therefore, distinctions in degree of authority in this area are not clear.

Individualization

Case management can individualize service by dealing with clients separately, assessing needs independently, and packaging services independently. Such individualization has several advantages. First, the best available (if possible) package can be assembled. Second, the easy route of institutionalization can be encountered. To the extent that institutionalization occurs because it is a ready-made package of service, that bias can be lessened by erecting a structure that will work to construct less-obvious packages of service in the community. The current informal and diffuse system, due to its multifaceted functions, is less attuned to avoiding institutionalization than will be the case management structure. Also, case management will have the resources of time and manpower to develop the more difficult noninstitutional-service packages. Finally, by removing the randomness from long-term-care-service decisions, we intend that ''better'' outcomes (less institutionalization, greater use of noninstitutional services) will result. Third, the perception of clients will be that they are being treated as individuals rather than being thrown into the maw of an insufficiently understood, complex web of a system. Individualization thus has both perceptual and concrete bases; client-specific review and coordination can occur that would counter the institutional bias of the long-term-care system, and the perception of this individual approach can have a symbolic impact that can reduce institutionalization. If a person feels he is receiving attention, he may respond more positively to providing the inputs of interest and energy necessary to avoid the often easier course of institutionalization. ''Whole-person'' attention can dominate a case management system.

Advocacy

Case management can serve an advocacy function, leveraging the system to make more noninstitutional services available. The advocacy is thus more system related than client specific. The advocacy will take the shape of "lobbying" for service, of working to elicit the best noninstitutional service the system can produce, and harness and package it for the specific needs of specific individuals. The advocacy notion comes into play if one considers that an institutionally oriented system is likely to need coaxing (at least) to generate adequate outputs of noninstitutional services.

Cost-Effectiveness

Case management can maximize the services received for the dollar by utilizing services in the most effective way. This factor is important considering the inevitable slow-down in funds available for health services. Also, it addresses the issue of "waste" as a political slogan. A lack of integration, real or perceived, is a political liability that feeds a public perception of incompetence in government. This public perception feeds back into the limited-funds notion because perceived incompetence, waste, inefficiency, an so on is not a good base from which to attempt to upgrade a noninstitutional-service network. Therefore, case management can be cost-effective by actually increasing the efficiency and efficacy of funds expended. It can also serve an important latent function of being a positively perceived government attempt at fostering competence. The individual-client focus helps; individuals can see a government entity serving them, not treating them in an undifferentiated "bureaucratic" way.

Follow-Up

An important case management function is to follow clients. Clients maintained at home must be monitored for continuing appropriateness of the service mix originally installed. Institutionalized clients must be followed to see that short-term, institutionalization-warranting conditions have not improved. Also, institutionalization precipitated by transient factors (for example, trauma caused by the death of a spouse) should not be made permanent by the growth of institutional dependence and loss of individual motivation and functioning. Continuing-stay reviews must be part of a case manager's role.

Case management can be structured to perform a variety of functions, ranging from minimal educating and "jawboning" activities to firm assessments, decisions, and implementation of individual service plans. The functions pursued are determined by the nature of the system, its needs and biases, and the type of commitment intended when the fluid notion of case management is used.

The functions are also determined by the answers to the questions that will be asked and the responses to the issues that will be raised later. At this juncture, it is sufficient to note that case management can be many things: it will perform a variety of functions, the functions vary in response to the system and to the implementor's desires, and case management can be "more or less" in terms of impact and influence depending on the functional mix chosen.

Case Management Program Design Issues

Authority

Relationahip to Service Resources. A case management system may:

Exploit current resources and exercise only the power to persuade,

Cajole existing suppliers and gatekeepers to provide better service,

Control and allocate service resources,

Develop service resources where services are inadequate,

Combine elements of control and persuasion.

Case management will inevitably have a role in the distribution of limited resources. Benefits will be as they are now, allocated under conditions of uncertainty and scarcity. A basic question is: Will the relationship of the case management structure to the rest of the long-term-case-delivery system be one of manipulator or decisionmaker?

Case management authority or prerogative is a critically important and tricky question. What is being considered is the case manager's *prerogative* to *control* the allocation of *resources*. The linkage is complex and crucial. Perhaps the key variable in a case management system is the extent to which the case management body exercises authority (discretion) to control the allocation of resources. Case management can function at many points between the poles of exercising moral persuasion and binding, authoritative decision making, and on this fluid continuum case management can change over time.

Funding. A case management system may:

Be funded as a coordinating device. If organized in this manner, case management would organize broker services using the existing system. Case management would rely on voluntary cooperation from service providers in this model;

Be funded to coordinate and purchase the required services from providers;

Make binding, nonvoluntary allocations but not pay for services itself. Case management could exercise a sign-off authority, controlling the flow of publicly assisted services through normal provider channels.

Service funding may or may not flow through the case management structure. Obviously, case management will be a vastly different entity depending on whether it must rely on voluntary cooperation to effectuate its decisions or if it controls the funding with which to buy the service packages (or controls their assembly) necessary to avoid or delay institutionalization.

Location

Location by Level. A case management system may be:

Centralized, at the state level;

Area based, by substate region;

Locally based, with a community orientation and identification.

Case management will fit differentially into the long-term-care-service system depending on at which level it is located. The relationship to providers, state officials, local agency actors, advocates, and even clients will be affected by this locational decision. It will largely determine the nature and tone of case management relationships. One cannot reasonably expect a case manager operating centrally to be perceived as positively or to be as effective with local provider groups as a manager based locally. Conversely, a locally based case manager cannot be expected to elicit coordination among state agencies on matters of service development and delivery as readily as one oriented toward state-level interaction. Physical versus organizational decentralization must be considered; a case management system may have central direction and still be area based.

Location by Affiliation. A case management system may be:

Free standing,

Linked to an existing agency or entity at any of the possible levels.

Again, whether a case management structure is attached to an existing agency or entity or is installed as a new, free-standing structure will affect how it operates. This effect will be felt most keenly in terms of likely success in dealing with various actors in the system. There are advantages to being outside of the normal administrative channels (for example, one is spared the pulling and hauling of agency politics), but such separation complicates the issue of working with the existing system, a necessity in a process predicated on coordination and integration of resources. The trade-off appears again—case management can be expected to be more or less adept at various activities contingent on its status as an adjunct or a free-standing structure.

Assessment Style

A case management system may focus on a:

Social worker model of assessment;

Nurse model of assessment;

Medical model of assessment;

Mix utilizing, for example, a nurse/social worker team.

Case management can focus differentially on the social, medical, or functional status of clients. The tone of the assessment will be very different depending on the assessment style. As the assessment model varies (and the concomitant staffing differs), so will the prescriptions that flow from assessment, the service mixes that are recommended, and the monitoring (follow-up) role to be pursued.

These questions must be answered before a case management system can be modeled or implemented. Clearly the answers to these questions will define how case management will relate to the rest of the long-term-care system and what functions it will perform. Different effects on the system and the possibility of performing different functions will depend heavily on the authority, location, and style decisions made relative to case management.

In the next section of the chapter we make assumptions about these questions to allow us to use one model of case management for the purposes of analysis.

Constructing a Case Management Model: Environmental Map and Service System

It should be obvious at this point that case management varies under different circumstances. A case management model can emerge only after assumptions are made relative to the status of the long-term-care-service system, the functions that case management is to perform, and the answers to the case management issues enumerated in the preceding sections.

The current long-term-care-service system lacks diversity of service resources and has its capacity largely in institutional-service settings. Capacity is understood to be the number of "slots" available in the system, the total volume of individuals who can be served, including all types of services. Diversity addresses the range of available service resources. The greater the diversity of the system, the broader the range of service options. As diversity increases, less dependence occurs'within the system on any one type of service (for example, nursing home care). The picture of current long-term-care-service resources that can be drawn shows a lack of diversity. The range of options is not sufficiently broad (see figure 6-1).

The long-term-care system appears to be severely skewed. A strong institutional bias exists in that most care is provided within institutional settings.

These service realities yield a long-term-care-service-system environment that can be "mapped" as in figure 6-2 relative to capacity and diversity.

Region 1 of figure 6-2 suggests a system with great diversity and low capacity. This configuration reflects capacity spread more evenly across services than is now the case. Currently, as figure 6-1 shows, the bulk of capacity encompasses institutional services. Region 2 suggests a system that combines diversity and capacity, a desirable state that has proved elusive in long-term-care services. A case manager in such an environment would work to avoid duplication and maximize optimal service mix; the case management function would be primarily a "traffic officer" affair, directing client flow to the appropriate mode of services. Region 3 posits low capacity, and low potential service mixes. We suspect that such environments do exist in undeveloped social service situations, but a system structure such as this is not an interesting or useful milieu for which to consider case management. Region 4 indicates a system with ample or adequate capacity but little real diversity. We believe that this long-term-care-service-system configuration most nearly approximates reality. It is the system map of the service distribution posited in figure 6-1—a system in which one service type (institutional service) predominates.

Case management has as its goal moving the long-term-care-service system to one that looks like figure 6-3 in terms of service distribution.

Such a system, by making a broader range of modalities of care available, would lessen the skewing that tilts the system toward institutionalization and institutional service. It alters the system to the extent that it moves the environment into region 2 in figure 6-2.

As noted, one version of case management will not be applicable to the range of all system features that can be found and that are indicated in

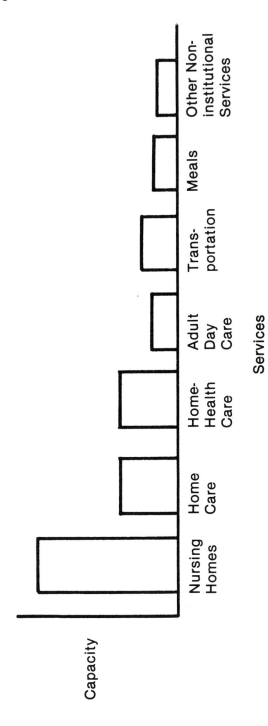

Figure 6-1. Existing Service Resource Patterns

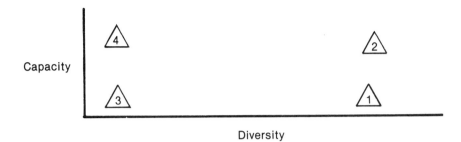

Figure 6-2. Long-Term-Care-Service Environments

figure 6-2. Also, no one form can deal with the very different service situations pictured in figures 6-1 and 6-2. The functions will vary in each circumstance and the answers to the questions raised previously, relative to authority, location, and style, must be different to cope successfully with the possible range of environments and service patterns.

Case management system structure, functions, and design issues are the basic considerations in building a case management system. This is the basic reality: Case management must be implemented differently to suit different environments and service arrays and to perform functions appropriate to each. The answers to the questions posed will depend on the system environment and the desired functions.

A Prototypical Case Management Model

To elaborate one model for the sake of analysis, we must specify assumptions relative to goals, system features, functions, and design issues.

The goals of case management, as it exists at region 2 of figure 6-2, are:

To maximize the use of noninstutional-service resources to delay inappropriate institutionalization;

To substitute noninstitutional for institutional supports wherever possible;

To alter the service components of the long-term-care system to counter the medical, institutional bias of long-term-care services. This alteration involves changing the service system from that pictured in figure 6-1 (skewed) to a figure 6-3 (diverse) situation.

The system features that are most relevant at region 2 are:

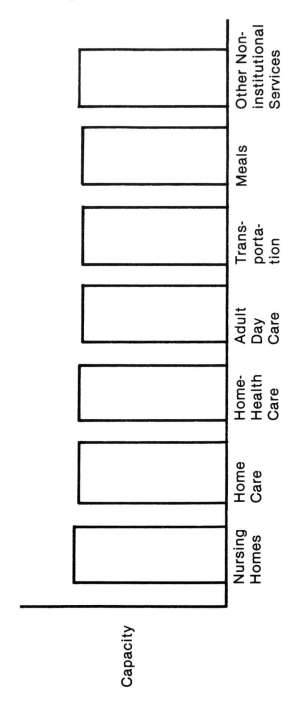

Figure 6-3. Desired Service Resource Patterns

Participating actively in the capacity-building process. Case management should not be equated with service planning and development, but we believe that in conditions of insufficient noninstitutional capacity, a case management structure must have as a conscious focus the development of resources. The role is somewhat schizophrenic, in that it combines coordination and development, but to be effective in the system conditions we posit, such a dual focus is necessary.

Identifying and, as with capacity building, helping to fill service gaps. A case manager is in a unique position to assess the effect the lack of a needed service can have—it can lead to institutionalization that could otherwise have been avoided. The case management structure must participate in filling these gaps, perhaps by presenting a strong case for the need, drawn from case records and actual experience with situations in which institutionalization could have been avoided. It is persuasive to say that x number of clients could have been maintained in the community if a given service was available.

The functions we see as most important at region 2 are:

Individualization, once diversity is to be sorted out and particularized;

Assessment, so that all possible resources of service and organizational support can be brought to bear to avoid institutionalization;

Triage officer, since targeting of services is crucial when capacity is inadequate. A case management system at region 1 must allocate within conditions of scarcity;

Advocacy, to make it known and increase the salience of the knowledge that capacity is lacking within the noninstitutional-service sector and that institutionalization occupies too large a place in the system;

Follow-up, to assure that only continuingly necessary institutionalization occurs.

The program-design issues we posed would be answered in the following manner for a case management model functioning within region 2.

Issues of Authority

Relationship to Service Resources. Case management will exploit current resources, but it must also control and allocate resources within certain parameters. The parameters of control are difficult to delineate; they can be neither absolute nor nonexistent. The system must negotiate the power it will cede to case management. Each case management development effort will be an exercise in bureaucratic politics.

Case management will make level-of-care decisions as a way to authoritatively channel individuals away from institutional toward noninstitutional services. As a by-product, persons requiring institutionalization will be approved for that service. "Matching" will be improved generally. If adequate noninstitutional services are not available, institutionalization may be authorized. However, follow-up must be part of the case management function to assure that institutionalization caused by transient factors (for example, death of a spouse, temporary shortages of homemaker/home health aides) does not become permanent. The case manager must be able to facilitate transfer when appropriate. A case management system should mix, in a negotiated fashion, tactics of control and persuasion.

Funding. Case management must be adequately funded to coordinate and have a staff capacity for client assessment, review, and follow-up. Manpower must be available to perform the capacity-building and service gap-filling functions as well. In addition, the case manager must control some funds with which to purchase service directly. This amount should be sufficient to close the gap between need identified in the client population and resources that can be tapped and funded through conventional means. In short, the more undeveloped the noninstitutional-service system, the greater must be the latitude of the case manager to act in that environment and procure needed services. The availability of funds should fuel supply to some extent. We must realize, however, that no direct-line relationship exists between funding authorizations and the supply of noninstitutional services. Many organizational, administrative, and political variables mediate the relationship. Therefore, the interface of case management to service planning and capacity building is important. It is beyond the purview of case management to replace the current funding network. The system cannot cut that broadly and deeply into existing arrangements and expect to utilize (coordinate) that arrangement. One cannot disrupt (or dismember) and simultaneously expect cooperation.

Issues of Location

Location by Level. Case management will be locally based in this model, on the theory that broader statewide operating effectiveness is less important than close contact with providers and community agencies, given the goal of maximizing usage of these local, noninstitutional resources. As we noted, a trade-off is evident. It seems more reasonable to choose the route that enhances case management leverage and credibility at the local level. We propose central organization and direction for the area-based case management structure; a central structure is needed to add coherence and consistent practices and protocols to the numerous local case management groups that will be needed.

Location by Affiliation. Case management will be linked to an existing agency or entity in this model. The advantages of "belonging" to the system in a significant manner outweigh the advantages of being a free agent. The existing system cannot be wished away, since case management is based on the proper utilization of that system. Since the system must be used, provisions must be made to work with and within it as effectively as possible. Being located outside the structure can foster an "us-versus-them" mentality, which often translates into unnecessary friction and lack of cooperation—two circumstances that are insupportable for a case management system.

Issues of Assessment Style

We posit a nurse social worker team assessment as the proper balance between a highly social or a highly medical model. The nurse and the social worker can and should educate the judgments of the other. Physician input can be sought as needed to deal with specific medical questions that arise.

In line with the assumption about nurse/social worker team assessments, the case management structure will be staffed with nurses and social workers, operating in pairs, locally, with the capacity to draw in other assessment resources as cases require.

We have now distilled our broad case management framework, with its myriad of possible permutations, into an operating model by:

Identifying goals;

Detailing how the model fits in the long-term-care-service system;

Showing which characteristics of that system are most salient;

Suggesting which functions flow most importantly from those system realities;

Positing answers to our questions on authority, location, and style.

The constituent parts of case management have been identified and the assumptions that yield one possible model have been made clear. Analysis can now be performed along a number of dimensions on that model (the "best," most "realistic," most "real world") to gauge its impact on the long-term-care system.

Framework for Analysis

The preceding section isolated one case management model from the range of potential forms. Assumptions were made relative to goals, system features, and program-design issues. The "model" case management system that emerged can be used as a benchmark to assess the efficacy and shortcomings of case management as an option for long-term-care-service reform. We can now consider the implications of making a unidimensional change—adding case management to the current long-term-care system.

We consider the potential effects of case management across a number of dimensions:

Organizational and administrative issues,

Political and economic feasibility,

Distribution of costs,

Effect on consumers,

Effect on providers,

Impact on service coverage.

Organizational and Administrative Issues

Case management is essentially an organizational and administrative response to the problems of the long-term-care system. It is posed as a remedy or, more realistically, as a treatment to problems within the system. It reinforces rather than reconstructs the long-term-care network. The basic question that must be asked is: Will it work? Other important questions are: Can a proposal that operates with and within the existing structure be an adequate palliative? Is the response made possible by case management adequate to the problems it addresses? Is the case management role inherently too weak or limited to strike at problems deeply rooted in system structure and practice? Is case management an example of putting an organizational Band-Aid on a systemic cancer?

The experience with pilot case management programs such as those operated in New York, Connecticut, Wisconsin, Washington, and Virginia suggests that results can be obtained from a case management intervention. These results are limited, however, by the size of the populations served by the pilot projects and the lack of coherent, cross-program-evaluation research. With this context in mind, consider some of the organizational and administrative variables with which case management must contend:

1. Implementing a broad case management system will be administratively complex. The number of actions that must be taken to

develop a system and the number of organizational actors who must be brought into play make implementation a cumbersome process. Pressman and Wildavsky note in their book *Implementation* (1973) that as more activities need to be undertaken and more actors must participate, the chance of success is lessened. As a bureaucratic/organizational response, case management must "play the game" within the current system to execute its mandate. Such an environment is not conducive to easy change.

2. Organizational imperatives are not unitary. The conflicting demands of the organizational and bureaucratic environment will create difficulties for case management. Case management must relate closely to those organizations and their members in its environment to perform its service-packaging function, and it will be difficult to deal with the conflicting demands and remain on good working terms with all the people who pulled and hauled on the system. As Allison discusses in *The Essence of Decision* (1971), organizations negotiate and come to conclusions about policy as an interactive process. It will be a challenge for case management to emerge from that organizational process intact and on speaking terms with the organizations on which it impinges.

3. As we discussed under issues of authority, a precarious line must be walked by case management between voluntary and "command-and-control" coordination tactics. Models that depend on voluntary cooperation alone will probably not succeed. On the other hand, case management is unlikely to elicit the needed cooperation if it is perceived to be an overly intrusive czar. This is an organizational challenge—to merge the power to persuade with actual authority. Operating under these constraints and negotiating with the participants to have them agree to abide by case management authority or to cede the case management structure authority will be difficult.

4. Case management must make and be able to live with an "average-personnel assumption," indicating that the program will be staffed and directed neither by morons nor superbeings. A case management director should ideally possess political skills, administrative competence, a familiarity with a broad range of program interventions and management techniques, and an ability to missionary. Realistically, the system must be able to survive with a less ideal director and a more average staff; it cannot depend for its survival on the consistent need for extraordinary staff.

5. We must ask whether case management will cause other coordinating mechanisms currently in the system to atrophy. It is a normal organizational and personal reaction to shed functions that are allegedly being performed elsewhere. The new case management structure must work well and utilize the existing resources perhaps in the form of receiving "official recommendations" from various points in the convoluted current

system. If the system does not work and present functions are shed, a net reduction in service-coordination capacity might result.

The picture is not altogether bleak. There are reasons to believe that case management can accomplish its function, in spite of or even because of its organizational characteristics.

First, the pilot projects noted previously, while not conclusive, do suggest that the case management of services results in less institutionalization, an expansion in the use of noninstitutional service, consumer satisfaction, and service individualization. We are not, therefore, embarking on a totally unknown course when we consider case management as a policy option.

Second, by focusing on the desire for formal coordination mechanisms, we may fail to consider the degree of informal coordination that already exists in the system and that can be built upon. Seidman underscores the role of this informal coordination: "We have created the false impression that most federal activities are uncoordinated. . . . Without informal coordination . . . the government would probably grind to a halt. . . . Managers who are motivated by a desire to get something done find ways and means of bridging the jurisdictional gaps" (Seidman 1970). The informal, random, ad hoc nature of the coordination makes it inadequate in itself, but it is an important plus for the development of a more organized, focused coordination effort. Case management is not beginning from whole cloth; important linkages are already established that can be embellished and formalized.

Third, an effort of coordination has symbolic dimensions that can be as important as the content of the coordination (Edelman 1971). Case management tells consumers of long-term-care services that their needs will be addressed on an individual basis and that the "system" is not a bureaucratic "black hole." A visible, approachable "helper" will be available. Case management tells providers that appropriate service will be sought, paid for, and supported. It conveys the impression to elders as a whole that assistance will be available when and if it is needed. The families of potential long-term-care-service users can come to understand, through case management, that a range of options is available for the care of their vulnerable members.

Fourth, for all of its organizational and administrative pitfalls, case management may be the least difficult long-term-care policy response in terms of its bureaucratic requirements. As it is the "middle ground" for cost effects, it may be the compromise position between making no change and attempting to reconstruct the entire financing and delivery base of long-term care. We must, therefore, consider the difficulties we have discussed in relation to the difficulties that would be expected from other options—options that might attack the current administrative structure root and branch. It may be more intrusive and difficult to implement a policy option that requires drastic alteration in the operation of other organizations (or their abolition) than to put in place a program like case management that requires marginal adaptations and changes in behavior over time.

We must draw several conclusions from this organizational and administrative discussion as follows:

> Serious questions exist about the efficacy of case management as a long-term-care-policy option—it may be an inadequate organizational response to a deeply rooted systemic problem. It may be an expression of a desire to "do something" in an area that lacks consensus as to what should be done.
>
> The structuring and implementation of a case management system will be difficult.
>
> Case management appears to have been a positive force in its limited trials.
>
> Informal coordination exists that would serve as a base and facilitator of case management.
>
> Case management may be the most practical response, organizationally and administratively speaking, of the possible range of long-term-care-service-reform options.

These conclusions yield a mixed analysis, suggesting both problems and opportunities. Such a result is reasonable in this area, since case management is so intimately linked to the existing organizational and administrative structure. This close linkage would lead us to expect complex, contingent interactions. Options that eschew the current structure do not face the specific operational problems of case management ("fitting" itself into an existing structure), but in by-passing the existing system and its structures, they may pose even greater dilemmas for reform.

Political and Economic Feasibility

Since case management will be linked closely to the existing long-term-care system, it must address the political issues that will flow from the environment. Only by dealing with the political issues can case management become integrated into the system with and within which it must work.

Case management is economically feasible. We can approximate the costs. They are not outlandish, and case management as an option is less problematic economically than other options that are more intrusive on the arrangement and organization of long-term care.

Politically, a number of issues must be considered. Many of them are the same concerns with which we must concern ourselves whenever we undertake a change. Some are more directly related to issues raised by case management. Let us consider some of the political concerns to which case management must direct itself.

First, case management must face the reality that politics can and does dominate over substantive issues in the formulation of policy. Lynn, observing a human service organization process in Florida, concludes that the key to understanding the results does not lie in addressing such substantive issues as the conflict between professionals and generalist city-managers or the debate between geographically defined or functionally organized services. Rather, the key is the political struggle "among actors with varying amounts of power and with different interests in reorganization" (Lynn 1976).

Second, coordination requires that an organization subordinate its purposes to some larger conception of the whole to which it is a part. The initiative for coordination arises when an organization sees the possibility of having another organization accommodate its wishes. As Rein and White suggest, an organization will resist coordination when it requires that its activities be subjected to oversight by some external body, and it will support coordination when its autonomy or power can be strengthened.[1] Seidman also addresses the point: "To the extent that it [coordination] results in mutual agreement or a decision on some policy . . . inevitably it advances some interest at the expense of others." The reactions of participants in organizations to plans for coordination (for example, case management organization will be inextricably linked to decisions made, implicitly or explicitly, about whether the participant and/or his organization stands to gain or lose from the change (Seidman 1970).

Third, case management is unlikely to become a serious issue unless a powerful political actor sees sufficient advantage in it to warrant sustained advocacy. Case management must be driven by an actor in the political system who will invest significant personal and political capital in its implementation.

Fourth, "bureaucratic politics" will be especially important in a case management reform because the reform is a bureaucratic response. As we have noted, case management cannot operate apart from the long-term-care system. It must be an integral part if it is to balance and tap service resources. The corollary to this reality is that case management must partake heavily of the bureaucratic interplay that accompanies organizational change. Relative bargaining skills, differential power resources, and interest level will largely determine the shape of the case management structure that ultimately emerges. As Lynn notes: "The precise form of the outcome will probably depend more on interactions—threats, compromises, and bargains—among actors with varying amounts of power . . . than on rational arguments (1976, p. 75).

Last, tensions are likely to develop among a series of different parties as case management is debated and its implementation is formulated. Health professionals will hold one view of case management and the role it should play. The operators of current provider networks will have a position. Established governmental health bureaucracies will have a stand, predicated on protecting their power and prerogatives. The case management implementors will bring another perspective to the issues, eliciting a series of responses from the other individuals in the system who have a stake in the organization and delivery of long-term-care services. Examples of such interested parties and their probable reactions to case management are suggested in table 6-1. The table is illustrative of the organizational reactions case management will spur that will fuel political conflict. "Health politics" will thus be added to the bureaucratic exchanges that can be expected. Entrenched health interests, in the provider and governmental administration and regulatory communities, will be wary of case management as a new political contender.

Politically, case management is complex and difficult. Integrating a case management structure into the constellation of provider and governmental actors will be a challenge. But, as with the organizational and administrative issues we discussed, case management is arguably more reasonable a change to implement than are other options. It is more practical, some professionals assert, to work through the organizational, administrative, and political issues posed by case management than to promote a change that requires the development of an entirely new approach and set of interactions in these areas. A definable set of problems exists relative to the political implementation of case management. This set of imponderables is far broader for changes that are not grounded within the existing system.

Distribution of Costs

Case management has a number of interesting cost implications. Since case management is linked to the existing service system, these implications are complex and contingent. As we observed earlier, case management is embedded in its environment. This close linkage causes the cost distributions and implications to be associated with the system realities of the long-term-care structure. The strength and weakness of case management as a policy option is that it is part and parcel of the existing system. It is not detached and irrelevant, but it pays a price for maintaining a connection. Case management must "integrate" itself into the long-term-care system as well as into the integrating services. The principal distributional, marginal, and total-cost implications are discussed in the following paragraphs.

A "cost of coordination" exists as surely as a "cost of regulation" ex-

Table 6-1
Projected Reaction to Case Management

Long-Term-Care Actors	Positive	Negative
Nursing Home Owners		Negative effect on cash flow; Limits acceptance of lighter care patients.
Home Health Agencies	More demand created, more opportunity for service provision.	Loss of control over client/service flow; Pressure to expand, agency may not be growth oriented; Uncertainty about relationship to the case management structure.
Home Care Providers	Same as home health agencies.	
Elderly Advocacy Groups	Focus for service to pass on to their members; Sense of more concern; better, more personal service.	
Hospital Discharge Planners	Case management can assist in shortening hospital stays and reducing Administratively Necessary Days (ANDs); Reduces pressure to find nursing home placement or arrange noninstitutional service.	
State Health Department	Better matching of client to service.	Loss of control; Question of relationship to the case management structure.
State Welfare Department	Promise of more cost-effective service delivery.	New organizational actor to contend with.
Area Agency on Aging	Build noninstitutional services; Better matching of client to service; Favored by advocacy groups.	New organizational actor to contend with.
State Umbrella Human Services Agency	Assistance in performing role of coordination and integration.	New organizational actor to contend with.
HCFA	Promise of better matching of client to service; Promise of more cost-effective service delivery.	Question adequacy of case management as long-term-care response.

ists. The dollar cost, both in terms of coordinating dollars and service dollars, increases as the case management structure attempts to coordinate the activities of more agencies and services. Therefore, the more "effective" case management becomes, in terms of the range of services and activities under its purview, the greater the cost is likely to be. The intensity of service search and multiple-service provision, when it is geared to individual need, encourages higher cost.

Related to this first issue is the question of whether case management can be simultaneously comprehensive and cost effective. Coordination is expensive as well as difficult and the cost increases as the scope of the coordination thrust broadens. It is therefore an issue whether there exists an inherent conflict between cost, in terms of dollars and necessary administrative and organizational resources, and a case management coordination/integration mechanism sufficiently comprehensive to deal adequately with the service needs of clients. The intensity of the case management function itself and of the noninstitutional supports that case management will prescribe may be very expensive.

The next question is: Does case management need to meet a cost-effectiveness test and, if so, in what terms? Should it only package noninstitutional services when the cost of such a package is less than the cost of institutional care? This approach, as it is being taken in New York, is probably self-defeating. Noninstitutional-service packages ought to be allowed to be as expensive as institutional care, on the assumption that an individual's being maintained in the community is having his or her preference respected. In addition, cost-effectiveness must be calculated in the aggregate, not on a case-by-case basis. The total case management experience must be considered, and it is not far-fetched to consider qualitative factors as well as quantitative ones. Case management holds the promise of matching services to needs, of avoiding both unnecessarily intense and unjustifiably inadequate service patterns. These factors constitute the effectiveness dimension of case management and ought to be considered with cost issues.

A cost will be associated with building a case management infra- and superstructure that can impinge on the flow of institutional and noninstitutional services. The core case management activities (assessment, service planning, service packaging, and follow-up) will require staff to implement them. The HCFA Task Force on Long-Term Care estimated in the summer of 1978 that a national coordination effort would cost $500 million for the add-on services of coordination, channeling, and planning. This administrative cost is real and must be considered if a case management entity is to be developed with any possibility of having an impact on service delivery. The following calculation suggests another way to derive a cost estimate for direct case management structure costs:

Number of events (clients processed) per year = 1 million
Amount of time per client = 18 hours
    Assessment = 3
    Service plan development = 3
    Service packaging = 6
    Follow-up = 6

Number of events per year × amount of time per client = 18 million hours

$$\frac{\text{Hours per year (18 million)}}{\text{Hours of work per case}} = 10{,}000 \text{ case managers}$$

Manager hours per year = 1,800
10,000 case managers × average salary ($16,000) = $160 million
Personnel cost ($160 million) × overhead (70%) = $272 million

If the assumptions embodied in this rough calculation appear to be reasonable, then the cost of building a case management structure may be less than anticipated.

Additional costs for service purchase (as discussed previously under issues of authority) must be considered. As we observed, a case management structure must control some funds to establish credibility, help fill service gaps, and allow truer individualization. If we conservatively estimate the percentage of long-term-care funds that could be channeled through a case management structure at 10 percent, we are dealing with an approximately $1.5-billion case management-funding pool. This money is largely reallocated, diverted from other funding streams, not new appropriations. Such a pool of money, controlled by state agencies and administered locally, would perhaps increase the efficacy of federal and state funding, on the assumption that funding decisions made closer to the point of service delivery are more efficient and result in more effective expenditures.

A second use of this funding pool is to foster the needed supply of noninstitutional services. Too many administrative, organizational, and political variables intervene between available service dollars and available noninstitutional services to posit a direct relationship between the availability of funds and increased noninstitutional-service capacity. However, the judicious use of discretionary funds can prime the service system to some extent, as an important complement to the organizational aspects of capacity building. The service-funding pool discussed here can thus both provide service to fill gaps and move the noninstitutional-service system toward the balanced image pictured in figure 6-3.

Although most of this $1.5-billion pool would be formed from reallocations of funds currently being spent on long-term-care services, we should realize that total spending will increase in the service area, if service gaps are to be filled and capacity fostered and built at the case management level. If we assume that 20 percent of the $1.5 billion is "new" money, in addition to current funding, we must add $300 million to the cost of case management, bringing the total cost to:

$272 million (personnel and support)
$300 million (additional-service funds)
$572 million

These figures represent an add-on of 3.8 percent to the approximate total $15-billion cost of the long-term-care-system in the United States. There are several considerations of relevance about this cost. First, it is a marginal additional cost. Second, some of the cost may be recouped by decreased institution utilization. Third, the case management system would be phased-in over a number of years so the cost impact in any one year would be even less.

Therefore, total system costs will rise (nominally) in a broad case management system. As discussed, add-on administrative costs exist. Also, the service funds will be largely, but not totally, reallocative. Federal and state costs can be expected to increase. Family-support costs could well decrease as formal noninstitutional resources are more thoroughly tapped. A case management system may wish to act to prevent too severe a substitution effect of this kind, perhaps by limiting formal supports underwritten if informal supports appear readily available and adequate.

The questions of distributional, marginal, and total costs cannot be considered in a vacuum. We have suggested that resources would be reallocated, marginal (administrative) costs would increase, and total costs would rise (nominally).

These effects must be considered relationally—that is, the costs are relative to current expenditures and other potential reforms. By the definitions we have presented, costs would be somewhat higher than under the current system, since an umbrella case management structure would be created and staffed and service and capacity-building funds would be made available. But the case can easily be made that case management is an inexpensive long-term-care-policy option. Major systemic change, affecting service structure, delivery, and financing, would be far more expensive. Case management, can, therefore, be viewed as a middle ground reform in terms of cost—more expensive than a continuation of the current system, but less costly than change that significantly alters the shape of long-term-care-service delivery. The proximate nature of case management is carried into the cost realm, as it was observed on issues of organization, administration, and politics.

The cost implications of case management are complex, but the basic reality is that it comprises a middle ground cost approach to long-term-care-policy reform. The costs are only marginally higher than under the present system and far less than a dramatic systemic change. The questions revolve around issues of costs versus results: Will case management result in service improvements worth the cost? How cost-effective do we require the system to be? Can case management be sufficiently comprehensive at a reasonable cost? Case management poses a basic question: Are the marginal expenditures incurred and the organizational changes required justified in terms of the pay-off we can reasonably expect?

Effect on Consumers

A number of advantages to individual consumers can be seen to flow from case management. First, case management is arguably superior to the diffuse and uneven "case management" function performed at many points in the current long-term-care system (for example, hospitals, home health agencies, home care corporations). The individual client currently may or may not receive thorough guidance, depending on the particular organization, circumstance, and even individual to whom he relates. One type of service provider may not impart information over a sufficient range of options—the view from one corner of the system may be myopic. A case management structure will not have tunnel vision and it will not have a stake in any particular service modality. Case management can assess client need and match services without regard to organizational interest, since the organizational interest is to improve client/service matching and see that, to the greatest degree possible, individuals receive the services they need. The randomness of current case management processes can be lessened. Uniformity in case management will improve client treatment.

Second, an assessment will be performed under the purview of the case management structure, which is sufficiently broad to consider all service options and which results in a written service plan, with connections to needed services detailed. Follow-up is inherent in the assessment/prescription/treatment continuum. This assessment, therefore, is more broadly oriented than assessments carried out now, and it has a sharper focus—to construct the most appropriate plans and to implement those plans.

Third, elders without family support are aided by case management. The educative, guidance role that may, in other circumstances, be filled by a family can be partially filled by a case-management structure. At the very least, elders without family need not go unserved because of lack of information. Also, service to elders can be fine tuned because there will be someone (the case manager) whose only interest is the appropriate matching of client and service. This motivation is not unlike what one would expect within a family. Family support can be made more practical and acceptable to families as helping mechanisms are made available through case management.

Fourth, case management should be even handled in that all who enter the flow with the same characteristics will receive similar treatment. The severely disabled who need institutional care, the mildly disabled who need a light mix of noninstitutional services, and the more severely disabled who have supports or attitudes of independence sufficient to maintain themselves in the community will all receive balanced treatment. Since appropriate matching is the operative principle, there is no reason to believe that any group, as defined by need, will be inadequately or differentially serviced. Arguably, those individuals needing noninstitutional-service packages function at a comparative disadvantage now—it is easier to address multiple need with an institutional response. Case management should redress this imbalance (assuming adequate resources and staffing) while still recommending institutional care where necessary. The key is that it will be recommended when it is necessary rather than when it is easiest.

Last, the level of general consumer information will be raised, especially when noninstitutional services are initially sought or when institutional services are sought for reasons of poor information or for the convenience of others. Case management may persuade seekers of service that a noninstitutional approach can and should be followed. At bottom, institutionalization will not occur without full consideration and understanding of the options.

Two issues can be raised about negative consequences of a case management system for consumers. The first issue is that case management may not be an adequate response as a long-term-care-policy option, since it depends so heavily on the capacity and flexibility of the service system. If case management is an exercise in managing incompetent or incomplete services, consumers may be better off with a system that makes more fundamental changes in service structure, funding, and delivery.

The second issue is that targeting of services may be weak under a case management system. The impetus will be to match services for all individuals, irrespective of how at risk of institutionalization the individual may be. This service matching will be a problem if case management is seen as being a mechanism to avoid institutionalization; it is not a difficult problem if this narrower goal is replaced by a thrust toward catching individuals earlier and maintaining functioning at a higher level. The emphasis—avoiding institutionalization or serving any segment of the population with need—will influence the approach of the case management system, and it will affect how different consumers are handled. One model will cater to the most-at-risk population, while the other will utilize resources to deal with those individuals who have a better chance of functioning longer in the community. In this regard, consumer need will be addressed differentially. As even-handed treatment is made available, specific targeting goals become blurred. Lack of differentiation in treatment can affect targeting capacity.

Case management is a consumer-oriented-service approach. Its aim is to individualize services, to match needs to services, and to provide individuals with the service level and type they need. Case management organizes information to consumers, assesses it in a manner useful for the implementation of noninstitutional-service packages, provides assistance in selecting appropriate services for elders without other supports, and is consistent in its approach in contrast to the possible discontinuity that can result from the operation of many case management locations in the present system. Consumers may "lose" in that case management does not in itself guarantee service resources, and it does not inherently direct the system toward a specific targeting orientation.

Effect on Providers

Case management will affect providers in that it will hopefully shift the distribution of service resources from an institutional to a noninstitutional focus. Within that area of impact, several more specific effects can be identified.

First, to accomplish its goal of utilizing noninstitutional services, case management must facilitate a "substitution effect," altering the service mix from a heavily institutional one to one that utilizes noninstitutional providers. The impact on nursing home providers, if case management worked as intended, would be to shift the lighter-care patients out of the institutional setting into noninstitutional alternatives. This impact is significant if one considers the internal-subsidy nature of nursing homes, whereby light-care patients "subsidize" the heavier-care patients, since the same rate is usually paid irrespective of client condition. The impact on noninstitutional providers would be to push that segment of the market to serve more people. An effectively functioning case management structure would stretch noninstitutional-service-provider capacity. That is why capacity building has been a thread throughout this discussion. Much case management activity, therefore, has the intent of inducing a greater supply of noninstitutional resources. Increased volume, from both new and existing providers, will be sought.

Second, to realize this substitution effect, provider behavior must be changed by case management. Strategies and incentives must be utilized to move the service system in the direction sought by case management. The case management-funding pool discussed previously is a prime mechanism through which provider behavior can be changed. The service dollars utilized by case management will reward providers who supply the kind of service desired by the case management structure for its clients, thus encouraging noninstitutional-service suppliers to provide more of the desired commodity. In addition, some funds controlled by case management will be used consciously to fuel capacity and supply. This control is necessary because, as we have noted, no direct-line relationship exists between fund availability and increased capacity. The capacity-building dollars can be used to deal with the intervening variables (for example, organizational, political, attitudinal) that block the relationship between demand and supply of noninstitutional services.

Third, changes in consumer behavior fostered by case management would be the final piece that affects provider behavior. As case management influences individuals to consider a broader range of alternatives and provides them with the information and the supports to effectuate their choices, different demands will be placed on the system. Both institutional and noninstitutional providers will be affected to the extent that consumers change their consumption patterns.

Providers are affected under a case management option by a number of factors. A substitution effect can be expected in service patterns, pushed by case management-service funding, capacity-building interfaces, noninstitutional-service upgrading, and changes in consumer behavior abetted by information and persuasion. The institutional segment would need to adapt to changes in its population and the noninstitutional-service segment would need to gear-up to meet the increased demand.

All of these changes would occur if case management meets its objectives of improving client/service matching, limiting unnecessary institutionalization, and maximizing the use of noninstitutional services. The purpose of case management inherently implies provider change. Reducing the skewing toward institutional service guarantees that both the noninstitutional- and institutional-market segments will be affected. Case management functions as a long-term-care-policy option only if these changes are effectuated over time. Therefore, successful case management, by definition, alters provider organization.

Service Coverage

Case management relates to long-term-care-service provision in three principal ways. First, case management must interface with the service-planning process to identify and help rectify gaps in the service system. There is no gain in coordinating inadequate or irrelevant services. Case management must be involved in the process by which baseline services, especially noninstitutional services, are established and improved.

Second, case management cannot be a substitute for clarity of purpose or adequacy of resources. Case management is insidious if it is used as an excuse for not developing significant service resources. Case management must not be a way to avoid addressing problems of social organization and human need head-on. One must ask, and be sensitive to, the possibility that "service integration" is a pseudonym for inaction. One can manipulate, view, and consider solutions to a problem rather than make the hard decisions necessary to treat the relatively intractable problems of difficult populations with which society feels it must deal. A symbolic, narrow, shallow response (integration and coordination) can replace a hard look and aggressive action directed at real problems of service organization, social commitment, adequate funding, and goal clarity. Case management must not be an "end-run" of commitment if it is to be a policy option for long-term care. We must not move toward a coordinative "solution" because the will to act and the funds to support action are scarcer commodities than vague efforts at integration.

Third, case management is useful relative to the coverage of services only if the linkages it generates makes the whole of the service-delivery system greater than the sum of the parts—that is, the primary utility of case management must be that it takes parts into a whole service delivery that serves individuals better than the system would if it lacked the coordinating focus. If the individual service units are not molded into useful, individually matched service packages by case management, its raison d'etre is seriously questioned. For case management to be deemed useful as a long-term-care-policy option, it must deal effectively with what are found to be real issues of service gaps, fragmentation, services, and programs working at cross-purposes, and individuals found to have multiple needs that cannot be addressed by a reactionated service system. If case management does not perform these functions well or if the problems themselves are illusory rather than real, we can conclude that case management alone is insufficient as a service reform.

Case management is relevant to service coverage in that, conceptually, coverage ought to be effectively expanded. While case management would not change the service array, since it is built upon the existing system, it should bring services, especially noninstitutional services, to many people who would not otherwise tap into the noninstitutional-service system in a coherent manner. Therefore, although the range of services and eligibility for services would not be changed, case management should increase coverage by increasing information, individualization, and service packaging. Coverage would be expanded in that case management would tap resources that might currently be available but that would go unused.

However, two limiting factors exist in this use of case management. First, the coverage is circumscribed by resource availability. Case management cannot make service available to individuals if the service resources are not available. Second, case management is limited in its coverage potential by its access structure. If case management utilizes a strictly central intake model, requiring all individuals seeking services to enter through it, a smaller system of services will be available from which to choose—as long as all funds are not controlled by the case managers, some service providers will opt out of a system that requires them detailed knowledge of the services available. A multiple access point system, which allows individuals to seek services from individual providers, again limits the ability of case management to influence coverage, because to the extent that existing provider networks are utilized in lieu of the case management structure, the potential for tapping all resources in an organized fashion is lessened.

Case management thus faces a dilemma: if it requires all service requests to flow through it, it might shrink the available service base. On the other hand, if multiple access points are allowed, the coverage engendered by control over client/service flow is weakened. One possible approach is to require central intake for anyone seeking nursing home placement but allowing multiple access if only noninstitutional services are being sought. This compromise is imperfect since only nursing home eligibles and interested persons are assured of case management education, support, and assistance. Also, the noninstitutional-service user is denied the alleged comprehensiveness fostered by case management. This preadmission-screening model of case management, which requires case management contact before nursing home placement, is a baseline—no one should be institutionalized before the full range of options is explored and understood. The issue of other, noninstitutional-service-seekers' being processed through the case management structure is more problematic. There are costs and benefits, in that comprehensiveness is advanced by central intake, but resource availability may be maximized by multiple access.

Finally, there is the question of private versus publicly assisted clients. If case management is to be truly comprehensive and add to service coverage, all persons entering the long-term-care system, or at least all those on an institutional track, should be "case managed." But the legal authority to restrict access for eligible individuals who are private patients is limited, even though a significant percentage of patients who begin to utilize long-term-care services as private payors very quickly become publicly assisted clients. This is an added complication to the issue of case mangement and service coverage; the greater the percentage of persons who enter the service system without case management activity, the less useful is case management as a policy tool. The ability of case management to impact the private-pay segment is questionable, yet this impact is critical to its overall success.

These complexities of resource availability, central intake versus multiple access, and private versus publicly assisted clients make case management an uncertain source of expanded service coverage. The long-term-care system is replete with these complexities and some professionals question how effectively case management can deal with the issues to yield real change. The problems are not neat. Therefore, case management is not an elegant conceptual tool with which to face the long-term-care system. It is a nuts-and-bolts, ground-up, bureaucratic, "muddling-through" approach. It should be understood as such and we should see the advantages and disadvantages of a reform mechanism that must constantly "dirty its hands" with the details of the system into which it is embedded.

Conclusion

Case management offers much as an option for long-term care. It can lessen the skewing in the current system toward institutional service. Similarly, it can reduce the medical bias within the long-term-care system. Case management can benefit consumers by increasing the responsiveness of the long-term-care system to constituent need. Case management can produce this result without requiring fundamental changes in the financing, organization, or delivery of services. Also, case management can contribute without exacting an exorbitant cost—as we saw, such a system would entail only a marginal cost increase that could be offset by the savings it would generate. Case management would reduce the inequity that marks assessment, placement, and service packaging in the current system. It would increase the effective coverage of existing services by more effectively linking client need and service. The long-term-care system can be made more "personal" through the use of case management. Individuals would receive unique, appropriate service mixes. They would have an agent within the system to function as guide and helper, and they would have increased opportunity to express preferences, note their level of satisfaction, and be active participants in changes made in their service patterns. Case management presents the opportunity for focusing the multiple points of authority and funding within the current system. Different forms of case management can be utilized to suit particular environments, pursue different goals, and perform various functions.

Apparently the desirability of case management as an option for long-term care depends on two issues. First, one must ask whether it will work. It is not certain that case management can make a sufficient impact across a broad-enough range of services and clients to comprise a full option. Also, one must question whether a large case management structure can be supported organizationally: Is case management administratively feasible when contemplated on a national scale or will it fall under the weight of its own administrative baggage?

Several factors affect our assessment of this issue. First, case management must interface with capacity-building efforts. It must rest upon at least a moderately comprehensive set of services; it cannot hold up an insufficient, gap-filled service system. The problem of supporting a large case management structure is lessened as the service infrastructure is strengthened. Second, our concerns may be assuaged by the fact that case management is primarily an entity to orchestrate services. As difficult as that may be, it is a less burdensome responsibility than elaborating the parameters and details of an entirely new intervention. Finally, case management models exist that show, on a limited basis, that case management can be structured, organized, and administered in a manner that positively affects the provision of long-term-care services. The Community Care Organizations (CCOs) in Wisconsin, "Access" in Rochester, New York, "Triage" in Connecticut, and the Medicaid Demonstration Program in Olympia, Washington, are all operating models with clearly established, detailed procedures and track records. These case management structures can lead us to believe that case management is a practical, "implementable" function. We have working models to observe; we do not have to guess about whether a structure can be developed, procedures implemented, and results obtained and documented.

The second issue about the desirability of case management revolves around one's view of incremental change. Case management is less attractive as one believes that other, more systemic options exist, are desirable, and can be implemented. One may conclude that a more thoroughgoing change is needed and possible. Such a conclusion must rest on a belief system that favors systemic to incremental change and that generates the will to act "radically" and the faith to accept the feasibility of nonincremental change.

Martin Rein observes:

> Every policy analyst must come to terms with the philosophy of incrementalism. His assessment of the ability of specific policies to cope with the problems for which they are designed will rest upon whether he repudiates, embraces, or comprises with the doctrine of incrementalism. [1976, p. 162]

One's values thus become the basic test of the desirability of case management as an option in long-term care. Either one accepts incrementalism as embodied in a case management structure to orchestrate the current system, or one prefers changes grounded in structural alterations of financing and delivery mechanisms. Predictions about feasibility, practicality, and end-results hinge importantly on the value premises that underlie the policy assessment and choice.

We cannot develop a common, universally accepted standard for judging the desirability of policies in terms of political feasibility, ideological comfort, and compelling rationality, since these decisions rely so heavily on personal policy-style preferences (incremental versus nonincremental policymaking). But we have seen that case management is advantageous along many dimensions and so it is a viable option, given the appropriate mind-set of the relevant decisionmakers.

Note

1. These notions are drawn from M. Rein and S. White. May 13, 1977. "Early childhood education: practice worries and the plea for coordination." Organization for Economic Cooperation and Development. Center for Educational Research and Innovation, Monograph.

References

Allison, G.T. 1971. *The Essence of Decision*. Boston: Little, Brown.
Edelman, M. 1971. "The Creation of Political Beliefs Through Categorization." Institute for Research on Poverty, Discussion Paper, February 1975; and Edelman, Murray. *The Politics of Symbolic Action*, Institute for Research on Poverty Monograph Series. Chicago, Ill.: Markham Publishing Co.
Lynn, Jr., L.E. 1976. "Organizing Human Services in Florida: A Study of the Public Policy Process." *Evaluation*, 3, (1,2):75.
Pressman, J.L., and Wildavsky, A.B. 1973. *Implementation*. Berkeley: University of California Press.
Rein, M. 1976. *Social Science and Public Policy*. London: Penguin Books Ltd., p. 162.
Seidman, H. 1970. *Politics, Position, and Power: The Dynamics of Federal Organization*. New York: Oxford University Press, p. 170.

7 Single Agency Option for Long-Term Care

James J. Callahan, Jr.

The notion of a single community-based agency for long-term care has been the subject of increased interest on the part of health policymakers in recent years. Various proposals call for a flexible community-based organization serving as a point of entry for some or all long-term-care individuals. It will perform patient assessment, provide or arrange for service, monitor quality, develop the system, coordinate resources, and improve patient care. All this will be done while controlling costs, reducing inefficiencies, safeguarding patient rights, and placing people in the least-restrictive environment. The rationale behind the single agency concept is that it will provide an identifiable focal point for long-term care, reduce fragmentation, and remove eligibility barriers. There appears to be an underlying hope that the existing problems of lack of access, inadequate resources, fragmentation, and high cost will be resolved somehow, if only some way can be found to incorporate all aspects of long-term care into one agency. Perhaps a single agency could resolve these problems, but one has to ask to what extent these problems are the result of underlying factors that have to date prevented the creation of single long-term-care agencies.

Previous Study of the Concept

A superb treatment of the problems facing long-term-care patients can be found in the Commission on Chronic Illness' study, *Care of the Long-Term Patient* (1956). The study describes the problems around coordination and integration of services and points out the importance of these processes for the long-term patient with his or her interrelated needs requiring simultaneous solutions. The study notes:

> No single agency in any community can meet all the complex needs of the long-term patient; yet without some central organization concerned with those needs, gaps and overlaps in long-term care are almost inevitable. The task of such a central agency is formidable because of the wide range in the needs of long-term patients, the multiplicity of ways through which care is financed, conflicting interests and pressures, the existence of outmoded facilities and other factors. . . . Chronic illness is everyone's problem and, by the same token, no one's clear responsibility. . . . For the long-term patient, the absence of a single responsible agency is a major lack . . . the individual does not know where to turn. [Commission on Chronic Illness 1956]

163

In the years intervening between 1956 and the present, great changes have taken place in respect to availability of funds, increase in the number and quality of facilities and expansion of manpower. What has not happened, however, has been a rationalization of services, better coordination and more careful application of resources to the needs of the long-term patient.

The single agency concept was revived by Morris (1971) with his Personal Care Organization (PCO) proposal. The PCO was seen essentially as a new organization within the array of community agencies. It would fill in the gap between available home-delivered medical services (Home Health Agency) and the combination of the medical, room-and-board, and social services of an institution. It was based on the assumption that a significant number of elderly persons became nursing home patients or lived a life of hardship because a range of needed nonmedical services was not available on an organized community basis. These services included homemaker, chore, home repair, meals, laundry, legal advice, and so on. Models were established in Wisconsin, and the home care network of Massachusetts represents an operating system based in part on the PCO model.

In the last two to three years, a single long-term-care agency has been actually recommended (Benedict 1978; State Communities Aid Association 1977; Correia 1976; American Public Welfare Association 1978) or discussed in a variety of options papers as something to be considered as at least a partial resolution to the problems facing long-term-care patients and/or policymakers (National Conference on Social Welfare 1977; CBO 1977; Pollak 1974; HEW 1974; 1976). U.S. Representatives Conable and Pepper each introduced his own legislation calling for the establishment of such agencies.

Certainly, the single agency idea is a bold if not imaginative approach to the problem of long-term care. As one reviews the concept as put forth by various authors, however, the intellectual task of conceptualizing an actual operating entity becomes formidable. Some long-term care functions to be performed by the agency are mentioned by all authors, while other functions are mentioned only by a few. For example, patient assessment is almost a universal function, while advocacy is mentioned only occasionally. This, in part, can be explained by the perspective of the respective author, but it reflects also a lack of systematic thinking about what a system is and how a system functions. The process of throwing out options in the absence of a conceptual framework fails to give criteria to choose between the "either-or" alternative suggested by various authors. What political, technical, and human criteria are to be used to select one alternative over the other? Will the criteria be the same in all situations?

The most serious problem in developing a national long-term-care policy is that no one really knows what the present system looks like and how it actually operates. The twin forces underlying the present public review of long-term-care policy, particularly the community-based support-services component, are the concern with the rising costs of nursing home care and the new awareness of disabled and elderly groups of their own ability to effect change and manage their own lives. The literature tends to be responsive to both of these forces referring to "alternatives," "community-based services," and the like. An ad hoc response to such pressures, however, while politically attractive in at least the short run, gives little promise of solving present day problems or leading to a truly better situation. Chapter 9 of this volume attempts to lay out an overall system approach to long-term care, which hopefully can be used as a way of looking at long-term care on a consistent basis, rather than on an ad hoc basis. This system approach will be used in examining the functions that a single agency will perform.

Models of a Single Long-Term-Care Organization

The comparative analytic scheme presented in chapter 1 will be applied to a single long-term-care organization. The problem at this point, however, is to identify the type of single long-term-care organization to which it should apply. Since a variety of functions are to be performed in long-term care, these functions may be arranged in many different ways as well as included in various different agencies. Models of single agencies have been proposed in the literature on social services, mental retardation, and long-term care. A brief look at some of these models will be helpful to our task.

Numerous models have been proposed to improve the integration and coordination of services at the community level through a single organization. Morris and Lescohier, after their review of service-integration projects, proposed two limited models that they believe may be feasible:

1. The most promising future lies in the direction of a *delimited coordination* which relies upon the following components: (a) reinforcing the existing loose network of service providers through improved information and referral mechanisms; (b) a limited external control over the flow of resources to this network, by empowering a central unit to reserve a marginal proportion of the total flow of funds; (c) the reserved funds kept within the authority of the central control, to be used to fill gaps and to induce agencies to reduce their rates of client rejection; (d) the development of a capability at the central control level to identify and monitor client reject patterns and service gaps.
2. The alternative model of limited *integration* would seem to be feasible for a limited number of publicly administered social services now scattered in several large bureaucracies with extensive missions. Some of these social services could be merged under a unitary administration to

carry out limited functions clearly in the domain of public service and complementary to the large bureaucracies from which they are drawn. [Morris and Lescohier 1977, pp. 41-42]

Aiken et al. (1975) evaluated five different models for services to retarded people, distinguished among three levels of coordination: a professional level, a program level, and an institutional level. They note that resources, programs, clients, and information are best coordinated at different levels. Resources are best coordinated at the institutional level, programs at the program level, clients at the professional level, and information at all three levels. This notion of different levels for the coordination of different activities is similar to that noted by Callahan in chapter 9. Aiken et al. and Callahan's three levels line up as follows:

	Aiken et al.	*Callahan*
Level 1	Institutional	System management
Level 2	Managerial	Operational management
Level 3	Professional	Patient management

While some differences exist, both authors note the idea that different levels of organization are required for the coordination of different activities. Aiken et al. have attempted to evaluate the effectiveness of different models to coordinate specific elements. The five models they discuss are:

1. Single organization with *some* services for a multiproblem client,
2. Single organization with *all* services for a multiproblem client,
3. Single organization with a wide range of services for all clients,
4. Coalition of organizations for a single multiproblem client,
5. Community board.

Pollak (1974) has examined the model of a single agency as the focal point of care for the long-term-care individual. He identified and evaluated four models. He assumed a situation in which federal-funding sources were combined, resource authorization was centralized, and consumers rather than producers were subsidized. The four models are:

1. Extreme centralization: A single agency does patient assessment, authorization, case management, and actual production of services.
2. Moderate centralization: A single agency does patient assessment, authorization, and case management, but services are purchased.
3. Decentralization I: A single agency does patient assessment and authorization, but case management and services are provided by other agencies.

4. Decentralization II: Same as decentralization I except that case management and production of service would be done, in most cases, by a single agency.

Two other models are also worth thinking about. They are:

1. A single federal agency model,
2. A public social service model.

The single federal agency model would involve the establishment of an agency such as the Veterans Administration (VA) or the Social Security Administration, with offices all over the country. *To minimize dependence on local service systems, it would directly provide all services under its own auspices, like the VA.* However, it could also serve merely a case management role. Such a national organization is probably not feasible at the present time, but it is a conceivable model.

The public social service model is similar to that promoted by the National Conference of Social Welfare and the American Public Welfare Association. Its features would include the following:

The local delivery unit would be the point of access (centrally or at outstations) to all the long-term-care services.

The local delivery unit would provide the full range of case-management activities.

All service resources that are publicly funded, whether purchased or agency provided, should reside in a pool or inventory available for use in individual case plans in accordance with the plan developed between case manager and client.

Each local public-service-delivery unit should have a certain amount of authority to choose the mix, quantity, and providers of services within its territory of responsibility, subject to existing regulations and possible requirements to use other public services if they are available.

The different models described here are based upon various assumptions. For example, Pollak's assumed situation was described earlier. LaVor (1979) has proposed an ambulatory chronic-care service (ACCS) as a means of improving delivery of service to persons with long-term-care needs. The model provides a set of principles to guide long-term-care-service delivery as well as some specific organizational forms. Its basic core entails ''the creation of an assessment and coordination function at the community level (LaVor 1979, p. 61). In many ways, it is similar to the model proposed in this chapter.

A Prototype Single Agency

For our purposes, we utilize a specific set of assumptions in proposing a
single long-term-care agency, against which we apply the analytic
framework. We assume that the present Titles XVIII, XIX, XX, and Older
Americans Act funding arrangements remain relatively the same, perhaps
with marginal improvements in the range of services covered and the
amount of funds available. At the present time, the financing mechanisms
for long-term care are very complicated. Both Title XVIII and Title XIX en-
title eligible individuals to a range of benefits that are paid for from an
open-ended appropriation. The range of benefits is primarily of a medical
nature. Titles XX and III (Older Americans Act), however, are based on
closed-ended programs that are capped at the federal, state, and even the
substate levels. Whether these are strictly entitlement programs or not has
not yet been determined by the courts. These titles are of a social service
nature and fund a wide range of services for a wide range of target groups.
Access to these services may be based on strictly defined need (for example,
court placement) or on a broad categorical definition (for example, over age
sixty). While the model we propose takes account of this fragmentation, it
would be compatible with a situation in which increased consolidation of
funding sources occurred.

The single agency would perform the patient-management functions
that, of necessity, must be performed near where people live. The functions
of outreach, entry assessment, certification, case management, and quality
control are compatible functions and would be housed in the agency. Actual
service delivery could be accomplished through any of four mechanisms:

1. Arrange for services based upon an individual's current eligibility;
2. Purchase services from funds available to the long-term-care agency;
3. Provide services directly with agency staff;
4. Combination of all three.

With respect to provision of service, disagreement exists as to whether
this would be appropriate for the long-term-care agency. The potential for
conflict was noted previously by Aiken et al. (1975). In addition, the Older
Americans Act prohibits the direct provision of services by an Area Agency
on Aging unless that agency was already providing such service or is the
only agency that can provide the service. This prohibition was written partly
to avoid so-called turf fights with community providers, but also because of
an expectation that the planning, system development, and organizing functions of the area agency would be incompatible with service delivery. The
actual provision of service, because of its immediate requirements on
resources, would absorb so much of the agency's time that the related functions would not be accomplished.

Another consideration around provision of service depends on whether the agency operates in a service-rich or service-poor environment. Schmandt, Bach, and Rodin (1979) discuss the implications of these two environments. A service-rich environment is one in which sufficient providers are available for an array of services to persons residing in the community. Even though they may not be sufficient to meet the need, the environment of need does have an array of agencies. A service-poor environment is one in which few providers or providers of only a particular type of service exist, and the needs cannot be adequately met. On the one hand, provision of services in a service-rich environment might be seen as duplication and could spur numerous domain contests. On the other hand, provision of services in a service-poor environment would be welcomed by clients and overworked agencies. Actual service delivery should be an option for the long-term-care agency.

A key issue is the degree to which the long-term-care agency controls entry into the system. Recognizing the plurality of actors and interests at the community level, complete control is doubtful and, at best, will be restricted to those to which the public sector has some payment responsibilities. Three modes of entry into the system could be selected. The first would be a situation in which *all* publicly aided patients requesting admission to nursing homes or other long-term-care facilities would be assessed on a *mandatory* basis by the long-term-care agency. Persons who entered nursing homes as private patients could do so without being assessed by the long-term-care agency. If, however, they found need to convert to a publicly aided program while at the nursing home, they would have to be assessed and certified by the long-term-care agency. Although it is conceivable that the long-term-care agency could review all admissions to nursing homes, it is doubtful that this power could be obtained from the various legislatures. Utilization of this approach would begin to develop some controls over inappropriate admissions to long-term-care facilities. For persons assessed as not requiring institutional care, an alternative community-based plan would be developed and implemented. It is conceivable, of course, that in many areas sufficient community-support services may not exist to provide the community-based program and prevent institutionalization. In that case, an ''inappropriate'' placement may have to be made and be recorded as an indication of unmet need.

A second mode of entry would be a requirement of mandatory assessment for all publicly aided patients living in the community who have been receiving two or more individual services beyond six consecutive months. This approach would identify those individuals who probably need some type of case-management service and who may ultimately be candidates for nursing home care. This early identification of potential need would allow appropriate planning to postpone or eliminate the need for institutional care in the community. The requirement that a person be receiving two or more individualized services for at least six-months duration would screen out short-term episodes and help to reduce demand on the long-term-care agency.

A final mode of entry into the single long-term-care agency would be the provision of assessment and case management services for persons with long-term-care needs who, on their own, requested such service. This request would be completely voluntary but the provision would be a service to individuals who wish to have some help pulling together an appropriate plan to meet their own needs. Some of the consumer organizations in the long-term-care field have expressed an interest in such a service.

The functions of the single long-term-care agency just outlined are at the patient-management level. Functions such as community planning, system development, evaluation, and the like are not included in this model. Theoretically, it would be possible to include other functions of the long-term-care system with the patient-management functions. We shall argue, however, that except in the case of large, departmentalized state or county structures, the nonpatient-management functions be performed by an organization(s) other than the one carrying out the patient-management functions. The reason for this separation is that studies have shown, and task forces have recommended, that planning, system development, and like activities are better off separated from service-delivery activities (National Conference on Social Welfare 1977; HEW 1976). Not only does a potential for role conflict exist but also competition for scarce organizational resources. While such competition will always exist, the separation of structures is a means of avoiding internal strain around resource allocation. Another reason for separating the two types of functions is that the geographic scopes tend to differ. Entry, assessment, and service delivery need to occur close to the clients and within a defined network of service agencies. Planning, system development, and the like, while incorporating the smaller geographic scope, can be done on a wider basis from the county level even up to the state level. In the case of the advocacy function, for example, to be effective it should have its own separate organization. Although advocacy is seen as part of case management, in the long run a case manager must become a negotiator for his or her client. Advocacy should be carried out by existing advocacy and legal-service organizations.

To summarize briefly, the patient-management function should not be incorporated with the operational-management functions, except in specific situations in which their respective integrity would not be affected.

Agency Types

At least five types of agencies might be candidates to perform the function of a single long-term-care organization. They are (1) Area Agency on Aging;

(2) the local Title XX social service agency; (3) local public health department; (4) local provider agency; and (5) special demonstration agency funded under Title XVIII, Title XIX, or demonstration funds. Table 7-1 is a very rough attempt to estimate the respective abilities of these organizations to perform designated functions. It is more illustrative than definitive and serves to point up the need to evaluate organizational capabilities around specific functions. As an example of how a particular agency would be evaluated, an appendix to this chapter examines in some detail the ability of the Area Agency on Aging to perform the functions of the long-term-care system.

Previously it was noted that services would be financed from current funding streams based on an individual's current eligibilities. The problem remains of how to fund the long-term-care agency. It is proposed that both Medicare and Medicaid reimburse the long-term-care agency, based on a rate established for assessment, case management, and related functions. The rate could be either a per capita rate based on the number of individuals who pass through the agency or the number of beneficiaries in a particular community. In addition, a certain amount of funds attributable to long-term care should be set aside from Titles XX and III at the state level. These funds would be allocated to the long-term-care agency to support certain nonpatient-related functions as well as patient-related functions for patients not covered under Medicare or Medicaid.

At the state level, a single state agency (new or existing) should be designated to be *responsible* for system-management and operational-management functions. Some activities such as licensing may be performed by other agencies, but the single state agency would develop licensing standards and receive data on licensed providers. The agency would have control over the percentage of Titles XX and III funds spent in long-term care, but Titles XVIII and XIX would operate as at present. The key to success at the state level is to give responsibility for long-term care to an identifiable, accountable agency.

At the national level, a new federal program should be enacted to establish a planning process that will pull together the long-term-care provisions of existing programs including Titles XVIII, XIX, XX, and III. Such a program need not immediately alter the existing federal agency structure, but it would necessitate the designation of a single federal agency to review state plans submitted under the program. This type of planning process could evolve into a more programmatic agency, which would ultimately become a funding agency.

Framework for Analysis

The common framework of analysis being used for the options applies to the single agency as discussed in the following sections.

Table 7-1
Estimated Respective Ability of Selected Organizations to Perform Functions of a Long-Term-Care Agency

Function	Area Agency on Aging	Public Social Service Agency	Public Health Agency	Health or Social Service Provider Agency	Demonstration Agency
Financing	Major funding would come from outside the long-term-care agency				
Planning	H	M	M	L	M
System Development	M	M	M	L	M
System Control	L	M	M	L	M
Evaluation	L	L	L	L	L
Advocacy	H	L	M	M	M
Information System (community)	L	M	L	L	L
Community Coordination	H (for elderly) M (for others)	M	M	L	L
Interagency Quality Control	L	M	H	L	L
Payment of Bills	L	H	M	L	H
Outreach	H	L	M	M	M
Entry/Access	H (for elderly) M (for others)	H (for poor and dependent cases) L (general public)	M	H (for specific service) M (for others)	M
Assessment	M	H	M	H (for specific service) M (for others)	H
Eligibility Certification	L	H	L	L	H
Case Management	M	H	M	M	M
Service Delivery (direct or contract)	L (delivery) M (contracting)	L (delivery) H (contract)	M (delivery) L (contract)	H (delivery) M (contract)	M
Patient-Information System	M	H	M	H	H
Individual Quality Control	M	L	M	M	H

Key: H = High, M = Medium, L = Low.

Coverage

The single long-term-care-agency option, in and of itself, does not expand coverage to more people. It does, however, provide new benefits to certain eligible long-term-care patients—namely, an assessment, development of a care plan, and case management. A result of this provision could be improved quality of care. To meet adequately all the patient needs identified may require additional benefit coverage, but this issue is separate from the notion of a single agency.

Access and Impact on Consumers

The impact of a single long-term-care agency on consumers has both positive and negative aspects. On the positive side, access should be enhanced for all long-term-care patients because a visible, identifiable vehicle for managing their service needs exists. People, therefore, should know where to go. The case management function would do much of the negotiating for the client and perhaps open up service doors previously closed. Individuals without families should benefit significantly by the assignment of a case manager. Horizontal equity—that is, giving persons with like needs even-handed access to all services or a choice among them—would be increased through the use of a common assessment tool. The fact that the long-term-care agency would be monitoring service should increase protection against abuse or neglect.

On the negative side, it is possible that access to services for the severely disabled, the poor, and persons without families could be reduced. These individuals tend to be the most difficult to serve or to find placements for, and as a result they may be avoided by the long-term-care agency. In addition, to the extent a closed-entry system is established, there would be less incentive for other organizations dealing with these patients to work hard and dig up the necessary resources to meet the needs. In effect, the total community effort being expended on the part of long-term-care individuals may actually decrease with the advent of a closed system. The reason for this decrease would be that the total resources devoted to this task under the long-term-care organization would be less than the sum total of the individual efforts that had been going on in the community.

Consumer "freedom" would be reduced where persons demanding but not "needing" nursing home care were denied such care. While horizontal equity might be increased, some individuals may receive a less satisfactory plan of care than had another agency prepared it. The single agency would be caught in the bind of trying to be an advocate and rationer at the same time. Consumer freedom might also be reduced because public expenses now decentralized would be aggregated at the level of the single agency. Costs would thus become more visible and subject to potential criticism and budget cutting.

Distribution of Costs

The distribution of costs between consumers and government compared to the present system would not change significantly. Total costs would increase, however, to finance the long-term-care agency. Administrative costs in all likelihood would increase in order to carry out all the functions of a long-term-care agency. The establishment of a long-term-care agency would not likely reduce the administrative costs in the existing system. Those existing resources would be diverted to some other purpose if their work load was decreased. The administrative costs include not only the direct payment of personnel, rent, and related items but also the cost of increased complexity.

The proposed long-term-care agency, with its variety of functions, is a very complex organization. Mandatory entry would require that all persons in a certain class go through the long-term-care agency. This requirement would increase complexity based on the number of persons assessed each year, the number of persons who remain in the system, the number of providers with whom contracts are written, the amount of change that takes place in a person's condition throughout the year, and the multifunctions required by the organization. This complex system could impose greater administrative costs in terms of reporting and billing requirements on the providers of service. The one value of these increased reporting requirements is the opportunity they present to aggregate and disaggregate various cost centers. Costs could then be assigned to purposes such as basic living, treatment, and social care and would become the basis for more sophisticated reimbursement systems, although, as already noted, aggregated costs could become targets for budget cutters.

Organizational Control Issues

Control over the services used would be clearly in the hands of the long-term-care agency, as negotiated with both the user and the provider. The user will certainly have a role in the development of a care plan, and some consumer preference will be present. Providers, too, will negotiate over the exact conditions and nature of the service they provide within boundaries. Of the three participants, however, the long-term-care organization will have the greatest control of the services used.

Determining where control over demand for service will be located is difficult. The long-term-care agency could dampen or expand demand by its public-information activities and its reputation in the community. To the extent that a mandated entry is used, demand could increase substantially, since a variety of referral sources that previously would have handled certain cases on their own would then direct the flow of patients to the long-term-care agency. Other organizations in the community might assume that long-term care is the responsibility of the new organization, hence they can just "dump" their previous responsibilities onto the new organization.

The long-term-care agency in and of itself may not be a good targeting device. It would have a general community responsibility, and it would need to respond to the demands of upper- and middle-income families as well as the poor. Unless some type of financial means test is used, it can be expected that a good deal of its energy would go toward servicing the needs of these articulate and knowledgeable groups with the result that less time and energy would be available for targeting. A possibility, however, would be for the agency to develop relationships with other groups that could target for the agency. For example, a multipurpose senior center in a low-income area could be a source for low-income-disabled persons who are unfamiliar with or reluctant to seek care. Appropriate working arrangements with such organizations would help open up the long-term-care system to the poor and isolated.

Effect on Providers

Providers would be very concerned about the role of the long-term-care agency, particularly to the extent it is based on a mandatory-entry system. The providers then would be dependent for all their long-term-care business on the behavior of the long-term-care agency. The author has suggested mandatory entry only for potential nursing home placements for this reason. If no additional funds were fed into the system, one can assume that total supply would not increase. To increase services in one sector under these conditions would require some other sector to suffer a reduction. Those agencies and organizations faced with the reduction of their "cut of the pie," could be expected to fight these decisions, with all the concomitant community publicity. The long-term-care organization would have the opportunity to determine the distribution of long-term-care funds by the manner in which they utilized providers. However, predicting the effect of these activities is difficult.

While a major goal of the long-term-care organization is to keep a person out of a nursing home, it is not clear exactly what mix of services in particular situations will accomplish that goal. Quite possibly a variety of mixes of homemaker and chore helpers, transportation, meal service, day care centers, babysitting services, and so on would accomplish that goal. The utilization of the mix will depend, in part, upon what services of that mix are currently available. If funds were available for additional services, the organization would have the opportunity to fill gaps and develop more suitable modalities to meet individual patient requirements. A change in mix, however, would have the effect of shifting demand among providers. The effect would be similar to the effect discussed previously in relation to shifts in services.

Political and Economic Feasibility

This model of a single long-term-care agency does have political and economic feasibility if it is approached in an incremental manner. The single agency would be limited primarily to patient-management functions. States could select from a variety of local-candidate organizations and adapt to local needs. Functions could be added as the agency developed its capabilities.

Political and economic feasibility would decrease, however, as a move away from an incremental strategy occurred. To cover the entire country immediately would require 600-2,500 agencies, depending on how geographically accessible they were to clients. The administrative costs of such an approach would be high and could reduce the amount of funds available for service delivery.

A single organization encompassing all of the long-term-care functions is neither politically nor economically feasible. Concentrating so much power and money in one agency at the delivery level will not be acceptable to powerful provider interests. The political visibility of such an agency would serve as a focal point for the dissatisfaction of consumers with the performance of the system. In other words, an all-encompassing single agency could be blamed for everything. (It could also get all the praise, but in this world of limited resources, this does not happen.)

Appendix 7A
The Area-Agency-On-
Aging Option

The Area Agency on Aging has been suggested as one organization that might perform the role of a long-term-care organization. Area agencies on aging are established under Title III of the Older Americans Act. They are based on the concept that the planning for services, advocacy, and service delivery should begin at the grass roots. The intent is to create a network of locally-based, responsive, flexible organizations to meet the needs of the elderly around the country. At the present time, approximately 580 area agencies on aging exist that cover the vast bulk of the population. However, some geographic areas and population groups are not covered by area agencies on aging.

The Area Agency on Aging is responsible for carrying out the provisions of the Older Americans Act. The Act was recently reauthorized in October 1978, and the functions described for the area agency include the following:

Planning services for the elderly through the development of a three-year plan;

Advocating on behalf of the elderly, including monitoring, reviewing, and commenting upon all regulations, ordinances, tax levies, and so on of local government;

Developing a system of services for the elderly through coordination and utilization of grant mechanisms;

Contracting for the provision of selected services;

Providing such services in the absence of any other provider.

The Area Agency on Aging is responsible for targeting its expenditures by insuring that 50 percent of the funds are for access services, in-home services, and legal services, with some funds for each service. While no means test is used and all persons over sixty are eligible for Older Americans' programs, the Area Agency on Aging is required to target to the near-poor, the vulnerable elderly, persons in greatest economic and social need, and Indians. In addition, 1979 expenditures to rural areas must be increased by 5 percent over the 1978 level, and a focal point of delivery needs to be established in each community, with preference given to senior citizen centers. The state agency on aging must also give preference to a local general-purpose government of over 100,000 population if one applies to become an area agency.

Note: This analysis is based on the system framework found in chapter 8.

An important consideration in looking at the Area Agency on Aging as the long-term-care agency is the fact that close to 50 percent of persons who have long-term-care needs are elderly. The Area Agency on Aging might seem a logical choice, based on this consideration, although the other 50 percent are children and nonaged adults. It needs to be noted, however, that the purpose of the area agency is to be concerned with the needs of *all* elderly people, not just those who are disabled and vulnerable. Since the vulnerable handicapped elderly comprise approximately 20 percent of all elderly, concern needs to be given to the area agency's role for the other 80 percent. The recent emphasis on advocacy functions in the Older Americans Act highlights concern about the needs of those who are not poor and who do not require long-term-care services. Advocate groups among the elderly apparently do not want the area agency to be identified as a place for elderly persons with frailties, handicaps, and limitations. Their concern is to project a positive image of the elderly, and some groups fear that focusing on long-term care would reinforce negative stereotypes. This focus would be an important constituency consideration to take into account in deciding on the role of the Area Agency on Aging as a long-term-care organization.

Potential of the Area Agency on Aging

We will try to analyze the potential of the area agency by matching up its presumed capabilities to the functions required.

Financial Resources. The Area Agency on Aging at the present time does not have the financial resources to become the long-term-care agency. The total amount of funds appropriated in 1979 for area agencies is $443 million, only a fraction of which is spent for long-term care. This amount includes $153 million for area planning and social services, $250 million for congregate meals, and $40 million for multipurpose senior centers. For FY 1980, area agencies are on a continuing resolution and funds will probably not increase over the 1979 level. It would, therefore, be necessary to expand the funding arrangement for the Area Agency on Aging. In addition, Older Americans Act funding is closed-ended, unlike the entitlement programs such as Titles XVIII and XIX, which are open-ended.

Planning. The area agencies have been in the business of preparing area plans for the past four years and have developed some expertise in this area. While the quality of the plans and their success at implementation vary significantly among area agencies, the planning function is one with which they are familiar and for which most agencies would have some staff and technical capacity.

System Development. Area agencies on aging have had some experience in system development in the sense that grants under Title III have been made available to support new programs and projects within the community. One good example of this experience is an area agency's providing front-end funding for a day care program that then obtains its regular operating funds from third-party payors such as Medicaid. Funding has also been used to expand and develop mental health programs, create linkages between health services and social services, organize specialized transportation programs, and so on. The extent to which these activities were considered as formal system development, as distinct from ad hoc distribution of funds to interested agencies, is something that needs consideration. As with planning, quality of performance varies among area agencies, and we do not know how the "typical" Area Agency on Aging performs.

System Control. At the present time, area agencies have little leverage over control of the long-term-care system or even the system of services to the elderly. Their main lever is the provision of funds for service projects. Some states require sign-off and review by the area agency for elderly-related projects that might be funded via the state agency on aging. The system-control function, however, is not a major attribute of area agencies at this time.

Evaluation. Evaluation can be assumed to be an appropriate but undeveloped function of the area agency both from the point of view of abiding interest and technical capacities. What evaluation does take place is around a review of particular projects funded and the extent to which those projects meet their designated goals. However, no systemwide-evaluation is carried out to any extent by area agencies on aging.

Advocacy. Area agencies on aging are familiar with the advocacy role on behalf of the elderly. Although the actual involvement in advocacy-type activities varies by area agency, it is a function that would be considered as part of the area-agency rubric. Most of this advocacy experience, however, has been directed toward other groups and organizations in the community in which the Area Agency on Aging is attempting to change behavior. Earlier in this chapter, we expressed our doubts about the possibility of an area agency performing the entry, assessment, and eligibility functions and also serving as an effective advocate for the individuals involved.

Management-Information System. The extent of area agencies' involvement in the management-information area is not well known but can be assumed to be a fairly minor part of their work.

Coordination. Coordination is a function that a number of area agencies have become involved in around elderly services and more generalized community services as they relate to the elderly. It can be assumed that the rubric of coordination and some technical ability in this area does exist among the area agencies.

Quality Control. (Community level) Area agencies on aging, by and large, do not have any authority for quality control at the community level nor do they have any technical ability in this area, with one exception. The one exception would be the extent to which advocacy and ombudsman-type activities could be considered a quality-control mechanism.

Payment of Bills. Area agencies on aging, for the most part, have not been set up to process bills on any large scale. They do, however, have minimal accounting and control systems in respect to grants presented to individual organizations. Billing by these organizations tends to be on a monthly organizational basis rather than on the basis of services provided to individuals.

Outreach. Area agencies on aging have considerable experience with outreach and information and referral programs, which could be considered one of their strong points.

Entry. An area agency could serve as the entry point to the long-term-care system. Area agencies in Massachusetts that have been grafted onto local home-care corporations do serve as an entry point for a variety of services. A similar arrangement exists in Pennsylvania, where the area agencies on aging serve as an entry point for a variety of service programs. If a closed system of entry was selected, however, area agencies might find themselves in conflict with their own advocacy role, as they may be required to deny benefits to older persons who could not thereafter obtain benefits from other sources. One advantage of an Area Agency on Aging's serving as the entry point for elderly is the fact that it may open up access, since the elderly could identify with the organization. The nonelderly disabled, however, may be reluctant to seek help from an elderly-identified organization.

Individual Assessment of Need. This function could be performed by an area agency on aging and is being performed already by agencies in Massachusetts and Pennsylvania, among other places, for certain home-care services. Experience with assessment for nursing home placement is minimal.

Eligibility-Certification Function. This function could pose a difficulty for the Area Agency on Aging. At the present time, no means test occurs for access to services supported under Title III, and the whole philosophy of the Older Americans Act has been to provide services without regard to any type of economic need. A number of the long-term-care programs that would be funneled through a long-term-care agency, such as Medicaid and Title XX, do or may have financial-eligibility limits. This problem has been addressed in Pennsylvania, where the Area Agency on Aging arranges the care plan according to the services for which an individual is already eligible under existing programs. In other words, the case manager tries to find a program for which that individual is eligible, from which the individual can receive services. Multiple eligibilities do, however, carry the possibility of gaps in service coverage. Some evidence from the Massachusetts experience indicates that the Area-Agency-on-Aging staff finds it difficult to deny benefits to one group based on financial eligibility, yet provides benefits to others under other programs.

Case Management. The case management function is one that could be carried out by an Area Agency on Aging and, in fact, is being done on a limited basis in a number of states.

Service Provision. The Older Americans Act prohibits the direct provision of services by an area agency on aging, unless that agency was already providing such services prior to designation or if it is the only agency in the community that can provide the service. There has been pressure recently to eliminate this limitation by law and permit area agencies to provide services directly. The prohibition was originally implemented in part to avoid turf fights with community providers but also because of a feeling that the planning, system development, and organizing functions would be incompatible with the actual delivery of services. The actual provision of services, because of its immediate requirements, would absorb so much agency time that planning and related functions would not be accomplished. Whether the services were actually provided by the staff of the area agency, or whether the area agency contracted with providers for those services, would require additional staffing and organizational capabilities for the area agencies. Many of them have had no experience in the service-provision area. Another consideration would be the strength of the area agency vis-à-vis other community agencies in terms of being successful in negotiating for the appropriate services.

Information System. Only those area agencies that currently are providing some type of case-management service would have patient-based records. These systems could be set up in area agencies, however.

Quality Control. (Case level) Area agency with case managers, however, have had some experience with quality control in that the case manager is supposed to follow up on the implementation of the care plan. The quality of this activity would be dependent upon the skill of the case manager and the amount of time available to the case manager to actually monitor services. To the extent that the same person monitors quality and manages cases, caseloads would need to be reduced.

The potential of the Area Agency on Aging to perform the functions of a long-term-care agency has been presented in some detail. Much more analysis is required before any final decision could be made.

References

Aiken, M. et al., 1975. *Coordinating Home Services*. San Francisco: Jossey Bass.

American Public Welfare Association. 1978. *Report on Long-Term Care*. APWA Policy Committee on Long-Term Care, Washington, D.C., November.

Benedict, R. 1978. "The Family and Long-Term Care Alternatives," *Public Affairs Memorandum Number 2*. Washington, D.C.: Administration on Aging.

Commission on Chronic Illness. 1956. *Care of the Long-Term Patient*. Cambridge, Mass.: Harvard University Press.

Congressional Budget Office (CBO). 1977. "Long-Term Care for the Elderly and Disabled." Washington, D.C., February.

Correia, E. 1976. "National Health Insurance, Welfare Reform, and the Disabled: Issues in Program Reform." Prepared for Office of the Assistant Secretary for Planning and Evaluation, U.S. Department of Health, Education, and Welfare, Washington, D.C., August.

LaVor, J. 1979. "Long-Term Care: A Challenge to Service Systems." In *Reform and Regulation in Long-Term Care*, ed. Valerie LaPonte and Jeffrey Rubin, New York: Praeger. 1-64.

Morris, R. 1971. *Alternatives to Nursing Home Care: A Proposal*. Prepared for use by the Special Committee on Aging, U.S. Senate. Waltham, Mass.: Levinson Policy Institute, Brandeis University.

Morris, R., and Lescohier, I.H. 1977. "Service Integration: Real vs. Illusory Solutions to Welfare Dilemmas." Prepared for a Conference on Issues on Service Delivery in Human Service Organizations, sponsored by the Silberman Foundation and the Johnson Foundation, June. Reprinted in *Managing Human Services*, ed. R. Sarr and Y. Hasenfield. New York: Columbia University Press, 1978.

National Conference on Social Welfare. 1977. *The Future of Social Services in the United States*. Columbus, Ohio.

Pollak, W. 1974. "Federal Long-Term Care Strategy: Options and Analysis," Revision. Washington, D.C.: The Urban Institute, February 24.

Schmandt, J., Bach, V., and Rodin, B. Jan. 1979. "Information and Referral Services," *Gerontologist* 19 (1):21-27.

State Communities Aid Association. 1977. *Report of Arden House Institute on Continuity of Long-Term Care*. Buffalo, N.Y., December.

U.S. Department of Health, Education, and Welfare. 1976. "Integration of Human Services in HEW." Washington, D.C.: Social and Rehabilitation Service (SRS) 76-02012.

U.S. Department of Health, Education, and Welfare. "Program Design Choices for Long-Term Care." Memorandum, Legislative Initiative Decision Memorandum, Washington, D.C.: Office of the Secretary, August, 1974; "Long-Term Care Services Legislative Proposal." Memorandum, October 19, 1976; "Memorandum for Long-Term Care Community Services." Briefing, Major Initiative: Office of the Secretary. July 1978.

8

The Social/Health Maintenance Organization: A Single Entry, Prepaid, Long-Term-Care-Delivery System

Larry M. Diamond and
David E. Berman

Dramatic growth in expenditures for long-term care services, surpassing even the growth rate for acute hospital expenditures, has become a primary focus of health policy analysis as we enter the 1980s. While the fragmented nature of the programs that provide long-term-care services makes any estimate imprecise, apparently between 1970 and 1975 total expenditures for long-term care went up by over 500 percent (Bernier and Quinn 1980). Despite this large increase, the problems of long-term care continue to mount. Three of the major problems are: (1) long-term-care services are not well insured, making these services a leading cause of catastrophic expenditures; (2) long-term-care services are too often provided at an expensive institution; and (3) the financing and provision of services are done in a fragmented way with dollars' being provided through health, social service, and income-maintenance programs.

Because of the latter two problems, the federal government has initiated a number of demonstration projects that attempt to coordinate the varied long-term-care services needed by the frail elderly and the permanently disabled. These programs establish organizations, often referred to as *channeling agencies*, that act as agents for nursing home, home health, and personal services. It is too early to know how successful these organizations will be. Perhaps, more importantly, whether these organizations are the most appropriate or the most efficient in providing care for the aged is as yet not clear. They suffer on at least three grounds. First, they deal with only long-term health needs. Therefore, there is little interface with the hospital or the acute health care system. Second, they do not change the prevailing financial incentives. Thus, the underlying bias toward institutionalization still exists. Finally, they are not integrally linked to one of the existing delivery systems—health, income assistance, or social services. Thus, what turns out to be valuable in the demonstrations will not necessarily become a part of the existing delivery systems.

Numerous attempts in recent years have been undertaken to assure more appropriate use of high cost institutional beds and to reduce unnecessary institutionalization. We have witnessed the introduction of homemaker services, the strengthening of the home health movement, and an increased emphasis on ambulatory primary care. However, rather conflicting evidence remains about the extent to which these alternative arrangements do in fact reduce the total cost of health services provided. A major problem with many of these efforts is that they do not link long-term and acute care and thereby do not provide incentives to encourage the substitution of appropriate less expensive alternatives for hospitalization.

One of the major questions confronting health planners is the determination of the most appropriate institutional base on which to build a more efficient and effective system of care. Major contenders are: general hospitals (which have sporadically tried to organize comprehensive care under their control for at least fifty years); physician groups; health maintenance organizations (HMOs); home health agencies; and nursing homes or similar long-term institutions. Each of these "systems" or subsystems, reaches the population at risk, but development of a more comprehensive, efficient, and coordinated approach would require major changes by any of these providers.

One such change proposed is the provision of long-term-care services under a fixed budget arrangement. The underlying assumption of this approach to long-term care is essentially similar to the general argument for capping the Medicare and Medicaid budgets. On the demand side, many reasons also exist for supporting a fixed budget arrangement, given the incentives to overconsume. With respect to long-term care, the potential for overconsumption may be even greater, since the services provided are quite similar to those purchased as part of normal daily living. Clearly, financial constraints may be an important element in long-term-care system reform.

Fixing the budget for long-term-care services has been discussed in terms of a bloc grant variation—that is, federal budget ceilings for long-term-care services that pool Titles II, XX, and county levels for the population over sixty-five. Recently, the idea of individual client capitation for selected social and personal care services was introduced (Meltzer and Joe 1979). Fixed budgets or capitation is viewed by some policy analysts as a mechanism to: (1) curtail the sharply increasing costs borne by federal programs for nursing home care; (2) facilitate case management and improve resource allocation in the long-term-care sector; and (3) introduce improved management systems and controls among long-term-care providers.

Little has come of the fixed budget idea to date, primarily for two reasons discussed in detail by Hudson (see chapter 3): (1) state fears that a federal cap would create untenable budget constraints in meeting current Medicaid obligations; and (2) the difficulties of public management of a system as complex and diffuse as the local network for long-term-care service providers. Indeed, the concern is that both the problems of waste and inefficiency and the lack of access to appropriate services might get worse under a state capitation system.

Recent evidence from managed system approaches to acute-care delivery suggests potential methods for controlling long-term-care costs which combine fixed budgets with improved case management. For instance, HMOs have been able to benefit from their ability to allocate services and manage clients efficiently so that savings have occurred in terms of decreased institutional care. By expanding an HMO's purview to include long-term-care services, we may expect to improve the HMO's ability to provide:

A coordinated and comprehensive services package;

Incentives discouraging institutionalization and encouraging community and home-based care;

Net savings to the system due to the substitution of appropriate, less-expensive, treatment strategies.

Similarly, personal care organizations (PCOs) have demonstrated that savings can be realized in the long-term-care sector through noninstitutional service substitutes. These findings support the notion that system reforms that combine a fixed budget with improved case management may be required to ensure that services are matched to individual needs rather than to reimbursement incentives under Medicaid and Medicare.

Such a perspective is the basis of a new variation of the capitation idea. Under this new capitation scheme, the target population is voluntarily enrolled and guaranteed a basic range of necessary medical, social, and personal care services through the designated provider entity. The label given to this provider entity, which is directly accountable to the population serviced, is a *social/health maintenance organization* (S/HMO).[1]

In this discussion, we will be referring to S/HMOs as entities that provide a complete range of social and health maintenance services, from acute medical care to homemaker and chore services. Conceptually, it is possible to separate long-term and acute medical care from any proposed service delivery model, and to view S/HMOs as a long-term-care subsystem parallel to acute medical services. However, by segregating these services, we forfeit some of the best opportunities for economies of scale, for substitution of appropriate lower cost alternatives for inpatient care, and for efficient and coordinated management of the entire gamut of social and health services for the elderly. Hence, the S/HMO model discussed here routinely includes acute medical care services in its purview.

This chapter reviews the conceptual underpinnings of S/HMOs and presents performance data from managed systems that appear to have the best potential to evolve into S/HMOs. These systems include HMOs and comprehensive PCOs. Major variations of the S/HMO model are discussed, including organizational, financial, and service delivery options. There follows a delineation of anticipated issues relating to S/HMO implementation, including organizational and administrative, financial, risk management, marketing, quality of care, and political questions. Finally, the anticipated consequences and benefits of the S/HMO model are presented along with an implementation strategy that the Health Care Financing Administration (HCFA) might pursue for testing the viability of the S/HMO as a major long-term-care reform option. The appendix to the chapter presents brief profiles of provider entities now working with the University Health Policy Consortium to develop S/HMOs as part of a national demonstration project to further test the viability of the concept.

Conceptual Overview of the S/HMO Model

Conceptually, the S/HMO has many similarities to prepaid group practices and HMOs. Individuals enroll voluntarily, a defined set of services are guaranteed, capitation levels are fixed in advance, and single entry into a defined care system is maintained. Providers who are participating have similar incentives for judicious use of professional services, particularly high-cost services. Like an HMO, an S/HMO is intended to foster health maintenance and the early detection and prevention of potential chronic, disabling conditions.

Beyond these generic similarities are several distinct and important differences. The S/HMO is designed to provide social and personal-care services required to maintain enrollees on a comfortable, stable basis in home settings, as well as acute medical care services. The S/HMO's raison d'être is to target such services for populations at risk of institutionalization, rather than to service a cross-section of a geographic population. By its very nature, it is expected that S/HMOs will include a greater variety of local providers for back-up, contracting out a substantial percentage of support services, rather than offering centralized services through office-based in-house staff. S/HMOs will be financially dependent on federal and state third-party payors for reimbursement of covered services, and hence must target their approach to these financiers, as well as to the general public. This approach is entirely different, of course, from employer group marketing under the dual choice mandate of the HMO Act.

The general requirement for the S/HMO is that it provide service to at least one population group at high risk of long-term institutionalization.

For the purpose of this analysis, the elderly are assumed to be this target population, though other younger adult or youth populations including the disabled, handicapped, retarded, or emotionally disturbed are equally viable target groups. All of the groups noted here might be further defined by either severity of condition or severity of need (for example, low income or otherwise lacking access to services). Eligibility to enroll in the S/HMO would not be restricted by income criteria but could be restricted somewhat by prior condition. An S/HMO could manage its financial risk by limiting its enrollment to be within certain case mix constraints. Another approach to enrollment eligibility would be the application of differential rates based on actuarial calculations of risks associated with certain prevailing conditions.

The S/HMO presents a consolidation through one responsible provider organization at the local level of these generic system functions: intake and assessment, case management, funds disbursement, referral and service brokering, quality control, and patient information control. Strong, centralized provider controls are placed in the S/HMO to monitor system performance, especially on the dimensions of quality and efficiency. In addition, the operational components of an S/HMO that set it apart from both the single agency option and general case management reforms are: (1) capitation through prepayment financing, (2) provider entities sharing financial risk, (3) contractual obligation to clients and third party funders in the form of a service benefit package, and (4) voluntary enrollment of a designated target population.

Capitation rates will be negotiated based upon current reimbursement formulas for service units comprising the benefit package, projected utilization, and projected size of the target group to be enrolled. It is anticipated that government funders will prefer to negotiate closed-ended contracts based on budget ceilings, while private third party payors will more likely negotiate traditional per head premium charges.

Currently operating HMOs and comprehensive PCOs are expected to be among the likely candidates to evolve into S/HMOs. A further discussion presenting evidence to support this belief is offered in a later section, "Major Variations of the S/HMO Model." The following section reviews the relevant performance information to date on these potential S/HMO providers.

**Evidence from Managed Systems Suggesting
S/HMO Feasibility**

Entities with the requisite management expertise and provider skills to develop into S/HMOs will probably include several types of private and public agencies now engaged in the provision of long-term-care services. Two types of entities, however, deserve special attention for consideration based upon their performance to date as managed delivery systems: HMOs with Medicare contracts and PCO demonstration projects. This section considers each of these entities in light of current evidence as potential S/HMO provider entities.

HMOs with Medicare Contracts

Currently, thirty-eight of the two hundred twenty operational HMOs have negotiated Medicare contracts to service the elderly. Approximately 46,000 elderly are enrolled in these HMOs, representing 6 percent of the total HMO enrollment. Thirty-five other HMOs offer Medicare buy-ins (part B of Medicare Supplementation contracts); 460,000 individuals over 65 are enrolled in these HMOs (Bernier and Quinn 1980). The HMOs with Medicare cost sharing contracts (Section 1876) are reimbursed on a cost reimbursement basis for parts A and B at rates calculated on the service area's average per capita client cost. One case, the Group Health Cooperative of Puget Sound, has a shared risk arrangement with built in cost savings incentives. The majority of participating HMOs serve as Medicare part B vendors at reasonable or usual and customary charges without such incentives or cost sharing contracts. At the current time, however, the Social Security Administration is earnestly planning for capitation contracts with larger, mature HMOs. Legislation is pending to facilitate such capitated Medicare contracts at a rate attractive to HMOs.

The data available on the performance of HMOs serving the elderly and the implications of performance on S/HMO formation, remain somewhat limited since: (1) the reports on home health care services and extended care services are limited by the nature of Medicare's coverage of these services; (2) the great majority of the elderly in these HMOs represent conversions from those previously enrolled, and are not new elderly enrollees from the community; (3) in only one case of the nine Medicare HMOs studied in any detail was it possible for a random sample of those enrolled to be matched and studied against a random sample of nonplan members utilizing Medicare fee-for-service providers [this was a three-year longitudinal study of New York City's Health Insurance Program (HIP)]; and (4) Medicare, until the enactment of the amendments to the HMO Act in 1976, reimbursed for emergency and nonemergency out-of-service utilization by HMO members, thus further limiting the service controls of the HMOs.

Eight major studies to date of HMOs with Medicare contracts have been conducted. Five of the studies focus on individual HMO experiences; the other three are comparative studies. Nine of the twenty-six HMOs with

Medicare contracts are represented in these studies. In four of the eight studies, comparisons are made with non-HMO control groups (Lennox 1978). The data made available by the Social Security Administration for these studies were claims for FY 1969 and 1970. As anticipated, every HMO studied shows lower rates of hospital admissions and lower lengths of stay than comparable non-HMO Medicare populations, with reductions ranging from 15-30 percent. Also, as anticipated, every plan studied showed increased in- and out-of-plan ambulatory physician utilization (in some cases these increases were dramatic, such as HIP) and increased home health care use. Use of skilled nursing care, among the plans offering this benefit, was mixed; some HMOs exhibited moderate increases while others exhibited moderate or dramatic decreases. Overall, most of the HMOs exhibited moderate system savings—that is, reductions in skilled nursing care and hospital utilization offset the increasing home health and physician care costs. Other HMOs, notably HIP, showed net losses because of an inability to control the increased number of physician visits (Weil 1976).

In a similar study, Lennox (1978) examined 1969 and 1970 per capita costs for Medicare populations in six HMOs and in matched fee-for-service comparison groups. During FY 1969, the six HMOs studied provided savings of just over $1 million to the Medicare program; one year later, the net savings rose to just under $2 million. Table 8-1 summarizes the 1970 findings of this study. Costs per capita ranged from $17-$28 lower for the HMO enrollees compared to the fee-for-service elderly.

Among the HMOs studied by Lennox (1978) and Weil (1976), those that owned and operated their own hospitals, nursing homes, and home health care services (principally the Kaiser Plans in Portland, Oregon, Oakland, and Los Angeles) showed the most dramatic shifts of institutional expenditures to ambulatory and home health services. A second group of HMOs, which contracted primarily with one back-up hospital, also showed considerable net savings and noticeable shifts of expenditures. The HMO group in the weakest position was the one that purchased services among a number of providers. This group included the HMOs that showed a net loss rather than a savings (Weil 1976). These findings imply that an independent practice association type of HMO may not have strong potential to become an S/HMO.

In comparing capitation rates, it is significant to note the wide variations present. Interestingly enough, the most efficient—that is, biggest net cost saving—HMOs averaged $490 per capita. The mean per capita annual reimbursement for all plans studied was $375. Note that these data reflect 1970 dollars (actual reimbursements today are therefore considerably higher). Recent information provided by the Office of Research and Statistics of HCFA are reflective of the increase; a recent survey of 17 HMOs contracting with SSA under Section 1876 reported a mean of $400

Table 8-1
Comparison of Adjusted Per Capita and Annual Net Costs of Six HMOs and Six Matched Medicare Populations, 1970

HMO	Adjusted 1970 HMO Annual Per Capita Costs	Adjusted Annual Community Costs	Members	Savings
Community Health Associates—Detroit	$422	$444	2,975	$ 66,104
Union Family Medical Fund of Hotel Industry—New York	547	575	4,408	128,862
Group Health Cooperative—Puget Sound	339	356	7,440	132,618
Kaiser Plan—Los Angeles	479	504	28,381	716,194
Kaiser Plan—Oakland	453	477	30,127	718,980
Kaiser Plan—Portland, Oregon	361	385	7,922	152,656
	$434 (mean)	$456 (mean)	81,253	$1,913,416

Source: Adapted from K. Lennox, *HMOs as an Alternative Mode of Care for the Elderly.* (Washington, D.C.: Urban Institute, 1978), table 2, p. 41.

for part B alone and a mean of $850 for the few HMOs contracting for parts A and B reimbursement. However, these figures represent a wide diversity of types and maturity of HMOs. In addition, these figures are merely suggestive, rather than conclusive, of what reimbursements will look like in another year or two (Social Security Administration 1978). Data on other HMOs, operating under second and third years of Medicare contracts, show a marked decrease in per capita costs, as size and service experience increase. The cost ranges for this group are $200-$300 for part B and $500-$600 for parts A and B combined. Note also that evidence suggests that on the aggregate, the HMOs have serviced a population that is at higher risk than its age cohorts in matched population (Roemer 1978).

Beyond cost studies among HMOs with Medicare contracts, no systematic studies of quality of care, enrollees' satisfaction, or marketing success have been conducted as there were among HMOs with regard to overall enrollment and service characteristics (Roemer 1978; Luft 1978; Donabedian 1969; Gaus, Cooper, and Hirshman 1976). However, isolated studies have been conducted of some of these factors in individual HMOs. The Group Health Cooperative of Puget Sound, which currently has a risk-sharing Medicare contract, did a study of its Medicare enrollees and found a high level of satisfaction with their plan. Pearson (1975) found that the presence of an intermediate care facility reduced the incidence of hospitalization and made possible a progressive patient care system at the Yale/New Haven Plan. Hurtado et al. (1972) found that at the Kaiser Plan in Portland, Oregon, the presence of integrated home care and extended care services significantly reduced admissions and length of stay among Medicare enrollees. Germane, Skinner, and Shapiro (1976) reported that slightly higher proportions of individuals received care for heart disease, high blood pressure, and arthritis in an HMO than among those elderly serviced in the wider community.

The limited evidence to date regarding HMOs with Medicare contracts suggests that, on the whole, the elderly enrolled in HMOs exhibit the same pattern of hospital utilization as their younger counterparts—that is, significantly lower admission rates and total days of care. Although other services, principally ambulatory medical care, have experienced increased utilization, the likelihood of overall net savings to Medicare and to enrolled consumers is high. Large HMOs, therefore, offer excellent potential as managers of S/HMOs. HMOs, and related managed health care systems, directly control institutional admissions, discharges, and costs and can ordinarily facilitate patient transfers to less intensive care settings. Additionally, they bring to bear significant management expertise, financial reserves, concentration of health and social services manpower, and an existing referral network for specialty care services.

One current problem facing HMOs is the strict regulations under Section

1876 governing Medicare contracting. The very large, mature HMOs such as Kaiser have no trouble meeting these compositional and size requirements, but most of the developing HMOs would find the requirements hard to meet. Appropriate waivers might be granted for a demonstration project in such an HMO to field test the S/HMO concept.

PCOs

During the past few years, several community care organizations offering single entry access to comprehensive personal and social services for elderly individuals at risk of institutionalization have been funded as demonstration projects under Section 222 of the Social Security Act. The most advanced of these projects include the following:

> Triage (Plainville, Connecticut) is a comprehensive home health agency offering health, social, and personal care services under a cooperative arrangement among seven towns in central Connecticut.

> Monroe County Long-Term-Care Project (Rochester, New York) offers single entry assessment and case management for individuals over sixty-five, regardless of income status.

> Wisconsin Community Care Organization operates in three cities providing comprehensive social services to individuals discharged from area hospitals and nursing homes.

Services are provided through Triage on the basis of Medicare waivers, while the Monroe County and Wisconsin projects are funded through Medicaid waivers.

This section reviews the preliminary data on the operations of these partially managed long-term-care delivery systems, focusing primarily on Triage and Monroe County. Of particular importance in the analysis of this information is the determination of the rate of substitution of in-home care for institutional care and the sensitivity of this rate to various financial incentives.

Triage

Triage has issued a series of operational reports that provides significant insight into cost and utilization patterns of comprehensive long-term-care programs. The Triage research and evaluation team compared Triage cost and utilization data with Connecticut elderly populations serviced through

Medicaid fee-for-service providers, New York City elderly serviced through the Visiting Nurse Service, and a cross-section of the elderly in Cleveland receiving home health-care services studied by the Government Accounting Office (GAO). Adjusting for age and sex differences and levels of functional impairment among the respective populations studied, and further adjusting for comparability of services provided to functional subgroups, the research team found the following results (see table 8-2).

The report notes the relatively equal balance of institutional and home-care costs, 52 percent and 48 percent respectively, compared with Medicaid's overall expenditure of 90 percent and 10 percent respectively for these costs. In addition, the Triage report notes that the availability of a broader scope of services for the target population did not diminish family willingness to share responsibility for the caring functions (Bernier and Quinn 1980).

Triage evaluation staff has calculated the institutional (skilled nursing) days saved and the net dollars saved for FY 1978 through substitution of home-based services. These data are provided in table 8-3.

The program is credited with saving approximately 81,000 days of skilled nursing care with an associated net savings of approximately $1,675,000.

Monroe County Long-Term-Care Project

Another source of relevant data regarding the costs of comprehensive long-term-care services is the intitial six months operating report from the Monroe

Table 8-2
Comparison of Triage and Other Per Capita Costs, FY 1977-1978

	Costs	
System	FY 1977	FY 1978
Triage[a]		
Per capita	$2,880	$3,400
Institutional care	1,500	1,900
Connecticut State Medicaid		
Per capita	3,660	4,500
Institutional care	3,294	4,100
Visiting Nurse Service of New York City		
Noninstitutional per capita	4,800	
Connecticut Project Sail (Title III-XX)		
Home-care programs, noninstitutional		
per capita		2,600

Source: Edgar Bernier and Joan Quinn, 1980. "Triage: An Alternative Care System for the Elderly, 1974-1979." (Rockville, Md. HEW, 1980).

[a]Note the lower Triage costs in comparison to other matched programs.

Table 8-3
Project Triage: Institutional Days and Dollars Saved, FY 1978

Institutional Days Saved

Prevented 365 days × 168 clients	61,320
Delayed admissions	19,995
Total days saved	81,315

Dollars Saved

Gross institutional costs (81,315 days × $30.00)	$2,439,450
Less average triage costs per client day (81,315 × $9.35)	760,295
Net dollars saved	$1,679,155

Source: Edgar Bernier and Joan Quinn, et al., "Triage: An Alternative Care System for the Elderly, 1974-1979." (Rockville, Md. HEW, 1980).

County Long-Term-Care Project (Eggert et al. 1978). Two-thirds of the Medicaid population assessed by the project staff were referred to home- or community-based placements; inversely, hospital assessments of an equivalent population resulted in two-thirds nursing home placements. The six-month cost for the project's patients was just under $1 million; costs for the comparable group discharged by local acute care hospitals were just over $2 million. Comparable per capita costs were: assessed by Monroe County Project—$3,242; assessed by Medicaid (acute-care hospital patients)—$6,911. These figures illustrate the importance of the assessment function in determining not only initial placement but also subsequent movement through the system. Assuming no difference in outcomes due to the placements, noninstitutionally based assessment is financially preferable.

Summary

The Triage and Monroe County data together offer a beginning perspective on current patterns of long-term-care expenditures among selected provider types and potential shifts of expenditures under alternative organizational arrangements. The number of relevant studies is small, of course, and variations in costs per location and resource mix per location have not been systematically controlled. The data, similar to the HMO data, are suggestive both of ball park per capita costs and of the potential nature of the shift in the allocation of health resources when incentives are operating that favor alternative types of care and care settings.

One might reasonably conclude that PCOs offer substantial promise as potential S/HMO provider entities. Most PCOs are likely to have established a good network of relationships throughout local health and social services networks, and their orientation is clearly toward the substitution of personal-care services for more expensive health-related services. The requisite skills and capacities for assessment and case management can also be expected to be reasonably well developed.

PCOs have potential limitations with regard to direct health experience, control of physician's orders and procedures, hospital and nursing home intake and discharge planning, and financial ability to absorb risks. On balance, however, these agencies, particularly those now brokering a wide range of services with some controls over placements and payments, must be considered strong S/HMO candidates.

Major Variations of the S/HMO Model

Organizational, financial, and service delivery variations are all possible within the framework of the S/HMO. For instance, the range of services provided, the relative openness of the system, the method of control of reimbursements, and the sharing of financial risk are all examples of areas in which S/HMOs have some flexibility in designing their system. The following section discusses the major possible variations of the S/HMO model.

Organizational Variations

A wide range of organizational models are possible for the formation of an S/HMO. Provider resources and expertise, the current configuration of the local health and social services delivery system, target groups and geographic boundaries, and anticipated service packages are a few of the many elements that will dictate the particular model most feasible for a given community. Significant variations from current long-term-care organizational forms are anticipated. Some of the essential variables that need to be considered in organizing an S/HMO are the following:

System entry: Single or multiple entry points?

System boundaries: Closed or open ended?

Organization of services: Available at point of entry or primarily through a referral network of contracted service providers?

Target service area: Neighborhood or wider community such as geopolitical or defined human services region?

Target group: Currently in the system or largely to be enrolled? Public or private? Higher risk or lower risk? Size potential?

Sponsoring organization: Public or private? Existing or new entity? Single corporation or consortium model?

Legal status: Corporate status? Acceptable for receiving federal grants and contracts? In conformance with state regulations? Composition of corporate board?

Location of the case management function: Who does assessments, care plan development, referrals, and follow-up monitoring?

Although a wide range of organizational options are possible for S/HMO formation, functional constraints argue against the viability of some options and suggest strong controls and precautions governing others. Variables that distinguish the different options include: open versus closed system, public versus private, nonprofit versus profit, health versus social service entities, and broker versus deliverer of services.

Theoretically, it is possible to imagine an open system model S/HMO. For example, a town human services agency establishes a nonprofit, private umbrella corporation that will enter into contracts with any local provider willing to deliver particular S/HMO services to the target population at a negotiated rate. The problems of appropriate patient management and operational controls in such a system, however, would make it highly unlikely that this type of S/HMO could be viable. HIP in New York City represents such a model of contracts with decentralized physical groups; its Medicare contract proved to be unsuccessful as it yielded a net loss to the Medicare program because staff could not control for out-of-plan use (Jones et al. 1974).

A full services brokerage model S/HMO including decentralized intake and referrals is also probably not viable; centralized resources permitting intake, functional assessment, and active case management by the managing entity are probably required. As defined by Pollak (1978), the highly centralized or moderately centralized single agency model can be considered to have the best potential to become a successful S/HMO, while the decentralized models would have the worst potential.

It was previously noted that S/HMO entities that are personal care or social service agencies are faced with developing dramatically new financial and operational management controls over the medical care system. Limited evidence shows that such controls are feasible and successful. For medical provider entities, a host of new agency relationships with personal care and social service programs and much broader case management systems are required. Though the cost risks might be more easily managed under a medical provider entity, these agencies will face organizational and developmental problems that are equally as complex as those faced by PCOs.

Public entities forming S/HMOs will likely need to establish new governing board structures, representative of both the clients served and the local provider network. Private entities, particularly for-profit entities, may also desire to establish similar structures. Similarly, private, nonprofit organizations will, in many cases, modify existing structures for S/HMO governance purposes.

Given the organizational characteristics required for S/HMOs and the caveats just noted, a more explicit list of potential provider candidates emerges. Potential candidates meeting these criteria appear to be: (1) current HMOs with Medicare or Medicaid contracts willing to expand the scope of benefits and the base population covered; (2) private or public acute care hospital systems; (3) large metropolitan-based visiting nurse associations or other home health care programs; (4) current PCOs in a position to raise private capital, expand their service base, and absorb financial risk; (5) existing health networks such as neighborhood or community health centers with home health and related support services in place; (6) public health departments or social service departments or agencies; or (7) private specialty hospitals or large-scale, multilevel nursing home complexes or chains.

New organizational configurations are likely whichever of these providers engages in S/HMO development. Consortia, separate subsidiary corporations, or new community umbrella corporations are likely responses to the organizational constraints inherent in S/HMO development.

An Organizational Typology of S/HMOs

Within the influences noted above, several generic organizational structures can be described along with likely provider candidates. A preliminary typology of these S/HMO organizational forms is presented in table 8-4.

Financial Variations

Financing of an S/HMO is essentially similar to the prepaid financing of the medical model HMO or a prepaid group practice. A designated target enrollee population is guaranteed entitlement to a given range of service benefits as needed, and the budget underwriting the delivery of these services is established at the outset through a per head or per group fixed or variable budget ceiling. Principles of actuarial analysis will determine the budget amount.

An S/HMO can be funded through a variety of financial mechanisms. The primary funding mode would be capitation and prepayment through capitation financing of a population currently funded through the govern-

Table 8-4
An Organization Typology of S/HMOs

Organizational Characteristics	Potential Provider Type(s)
Single entry point for assessment; basic health, social, and personal services provided through an extensive provider referral network.	PCOs; related types of home care organizations.
Single entry point; comprehensive range of services available at a central site with personal care and nursing home services through contracted providers.	Closed panel HMO or chronic disease hospitals; acute-care hospitals.
Multiple entry points; assessment done on a decentralized basis; each of the intake sites provides a core of health and social services, with other specialty health or personal care services available through contracted providers.	Community health or social services center networks.
Multiple entry points for comprehensive assessments and limited health and social services; most services provided through contracted providers.	Home care networks; decentralized PCOs; visiting nurse associations; independent practice association (IPA) types of HMOs.

ment or other third parties, adding appropriate program waivers to cover the proposed range of service benefits. This might involve single or multiple public third party buy-ins. A second source of funds for the S/HMO is private payments, typically in the form of premiums, or copayments and deductibles to private grants or contracts that could support special needs not covered by other funding sources. These monies could be targeted for such activities as management system support, assessment instrumentation development, or operations support.

Outside grant and contract monies could also assist the S/HMO in keeping the capitation fee at a more affordable level both to individuals and to third party funders. Such additional outside funds might also include continued fee-for-service third party billing during the transition phase, to buffer the provider against the sudden shift to capitation financing. However, once S/HMOs are operational, they should be able to support themselves without depending on outside assistance.

S/HMOs might implement three major potential capitation variations: (1) a sum negotiated with a given government payor (for example, Medicare) to service a population now covered by that or related public programs; (2) mixed capitation models in which enrollees, currently covered by more than one program for services defined in the S/HMO benefits package, are covered through pooled capitation (for example, Medicaid and Title XX); and (3) populations potentially vulnerable to long-term-care needs, now covered through private insurance plans, could add on coverage to additional premium costs for S/HMO services (for example, a personal and social services rider to existing medical coverage). The type of capitation utilized will depend upon the target population in question and, in particular, whether a closed- or open-ended contract is negotiated by the third party payor.

Prepayment cash flow mechanisms will also differ among various funders and enrollee groups. Private insurers and Medicare will likely retain current monthly or quarterly premium collections and turn advance payments to the S/HMO entity accordingly. Other government payors including Medicaid, Title XX, Vocational Rehabilitation, and the Administration on Aging might instead provide longer-range lump sum payments such as annual prepaid contracts with the S/HMO. These variations in prepayment modes and corresponding cash flow mechanisms will be important variables guiding S/HMO marketing to selected enrollee populations.

The financial viability of an S/HMO will partly depend on the proportion of severely impaired cases in its case mix. Eligibility to enroll in an S/HMO may have to be restricted somewhat by prior condition. Persons with especially poor health status, for example, might not be allowed to enroll at a particular point in time unless the overall projected case mix allowed for absorbing such individuals, or differential rates could be charged based on prevailing conditions.

The S/HMO then will service a population that includes well, ambulatory, and mildly impaired elderly not at high risk of institutionalization, coupled with older and more severely impaired elderly. By selecting a target group that spans a wide range of conditions and needs, costs can be more easily spread across the enrollee population, yielding a potential pool of funds to absorb the additional costs of the most vulnerable enrollees.

Service Variations

S/HMOs are expected to vary somewhat in the service packages that they develop and offer to their clientele. Conceptually, S/HMOs could offer only long-term-care in order to supplement acute-care services received through a parallel system. However, this discussion assumes that the preferred S/HMO service delivery model would include both long-term-care and acute-care services, in order to minimize administrative costs, allow for economies of scale, and improve continuity of care and patient management.

The specific service package offered by an S/HMO can be expected to vary within reasonable constraints. The variation will be based on the availability of local providers and other competitive resources; the needs of the target population group; the size, maturity, and philosophy of the S/HMO provider entity; and federal, state, and private payor financing negotiations. At a minimum, the S/HMO is expected to offer a benefits package for the elderly that is congruent with the core services now funded through Medicare, Medicaid, and Title XX. At a minimum such a package would likely include the following services:

Acute inpatient care,

Inpatient and outpatient diagnostic and treatment services including all ancillary services,

Outpatient medical services including triage, physician and nurse visits, and social services visits,

Therapeutic services including health services, physical and occupational therapy,

Skilled nursing home services,

Home health services (provided either by visiting nurses or home health aides),

Optometry services and appliances,

Homemaker and chore services,

Prescription drugs,

Counselling,

Emergency mental health services,

Transportation services.

Major Issues Relating to the Establishment of S/HMOs

Given the complexity and risks inherent to S/HMO development, a variety of issues can be expected to arise. This section notes the major anticipated questions in the areas of organization and administration, financing and risk management, marketing, quality of care, and anticipated political obstacles. The discussion further offers a range of ideas that addresses these questions and issues, to help make the S/HMO concept attractive to potential provider entities.

Organizational and Administrative Issues

Similar to the other organizational long-term-care options under consideration, system management under an S/HMO delivery network would remain
largely with external agencies. Funding would primarily reside with state
and federal agencies; regulatory controls would reside at the state level; and
planning and evaluation activities would continue at the area, state, and
federal levels. Cooperative arrangements with funding, regulatory, and
planning agencies would have to be developed and maintained to assure efficient system management for the S/HMO.

For example, several administrative tasks are required for state, federal,
or private funders to assure that an S/HMO meets current regulations and
related program criteria. State Medicaid regulations governing provider
eligibility for third party payments to an S/HMO will need to be examined.
Extensive Medicaid and Medicare program waivers will be required. States
would need to request and oversee such waivers.

State insurance regulations governing the reimbursement of various services under the auspices of various providers, as well as general insurance
licensure requirements, would similarly require examination. Licensing and
certification of S/HMO providers and their facilities represent another area
for review and consideration. State certificate-of-need laws would similarly
impact on the S/HMO. In the face of current funding, planning, and
regulatory requirements, S/HMOs would need priority treatment as federal
demonstration projects in order to avoid entrapment in these administrative
obstacles posed.

As previously mentioned, new organizational configurations will be required. New boards to represent the enrollees, the providers, public officials, and the community at large must be established. In addition, a
cooperative network of providers in the form of a consortium, umbrella
corporation, or other model must be developed.

Of particular importance is the development of incentives for the
medical providers in the S/HMO service network, especially in cases in
which a nonmedical provider entity forms an S/HMO. Successful negotiations with potential participating physicians regarding marketing assistance,
rates, screening and triage functions, referrals procedures, orders, and
reports are critical.

Whether core S/HMO physicians, contracted community-based physicians, or some balance of the two optimizes both cost-effectiveness and
enrollee marketing potential remains to be tested. The S/HMO will attempt
to negotiate physician incentives that are better than current fee-for-service
Medicare and Medicaid arrangements.

Another important issue facing S/HMOs, especially nonmedically based S/HMOs, is the establishment of referral agreement with local hospitals and nursing homes. Bed guarantees at negotiated rates, particularly rates that could bypass transfer problems and revenue loss due to administratively unnecessary days, could be appealing to these institutions. In negotiating agreements with selected institutions, S/HMOs might successfully achieve discounted rates if enrollments grow to a sufficient size, similar to HMO negotiating strategies.

Finally, S/HMOs must administratively establish methods to allocate nonprofessional services such as homemaker or chore services. Rationing, copayments, queues, or other forms of allocation must be established in order to prevent the overuse of these services by selected individuals. In addition, incentives must be created so that the S/HMO does not provide home-based services when family members or friends are available. The substitution of S/HMO services for informal services already being rendered is not a desirable outcome, but it may be difficult to control.

Financial and Risk Management Issues

An S/HMO must address a variety of important problems that relate to financial management and the sharing of risk. These concerns directly affect proposed capitation rates, enrollment strategies, quality-control measures, and utilization-control mechanisms.

A basic concern to a developing S/HMO is the minimum size of the enrolled population needed to produce revenues sufficient to spread the financial risks. Medical model HMOs operate on assumptions of critical size based upon the realization of economies of scale and self-sufficiency once a target threshold is passed. For most developing HMOs this threshold is considered to be around 20,000-25,000 enrollees. This size guarantees sufficient spreading of risk, stable cash flow, stable loan payback, and most efficient use of ambulatory care center space.

S/HMO provider entities will be limited in size by the capture potential of smaller target populations; by lack of provider marketing expertise and resources; by the willingness of local providers, especially physicians, to participate in a major way in an unproven enterprise; and by enrollee concerns about being locked into an untested system.

Currently, among HMOs with Medicare contracts, the enrollments range from 2,000 to 80,000 Medicare eligibles, with most programs at 5,000 to 12,000. Among PCOs, the usual size range is 2,000 to 5,000 Medicare eligibles. What the minimum size requirements will be for an S/HMO is difficult to predict. The number of enrollees needed to sufficiently disperse financial risk will partially depend on where the system can produce efficiencies. This may be possible with smaller enrollments than HMOs, because S/HMOs may not have to rely on achieving cost savings through the control of utilization of acute-care specialists. Rather, economies are expected to be derived from the substitution of home-based care for nursing home care and nursing home care for hospital care. Perhaps a good penetration rate such as 10 percent or more of the eligible population might be a reasonable S/HMO start-up goal.

As previously defined, the basic package of S/HMO services was estimated to cost $2,500 per capita during FY 1977 for persons over sixty-five, on a fee-for-service basis across government programs (Social Security Administration 1978). Of course, inflation in the health-care sector has risen more than a third since that time and at current prices the S/HMO benefits package suggested here would likely require about $3,500-$4,000 capitation. The S/HMO would strive to market the service package to public third party payors at a per capita cost equal to or less than the current per capita amount, while simultaneously reducing, where possible, the amount of copayments and deductibles charged to enrollees.

Besides developing adequate demand for program services in order to generate sufficient revenues and financial viability, an S/HMO must also address questions of risk management. An S/HMO provider entity assumes risk initially by agreeing to serve a population that includes a percentage of enrollees at high risk of institutionalization at a fixed price. This risk includes not only financial risk but also organizational credibility. A provider entity that fails in the development of an S/HMO may be hard-pressed to retain a significant role in the local long-term-care network.

Given the possibility of unforeseen and uncontrolled events among a population enrolled in an S/HMO, a significant share of the risk must also initially be assumed by public third party payors. Shared risk strategies must be developed between the S/HMO and its funding sources, which include reinsurance arrangements for the provider entity and financial reserves. However, if provider negligence such as inadequate utilization of case mix controls, is demonstrated, the S/HMO cannot avoid assuming portions of risk incurred beyond the capitated budget ceiling. In addition, providers are anticipated to assume greater portions of overall risk once the S/HMO has stabilized.

To implement the shared risk concept, specified financial requirements will need to be negotiated by an S/HMO. S/HMOs will be required to maintain a level of financial reserves (bonding or escrow accounts) and to execute reinsurance agreements with the support of its funding sources. Private provider entities assuming S/HMO responsibility, either directly or by subcontract, will negotiate the specific stockholder or partner risks to be assumed. Similarly, persons serving on the boards of S/HMOs must realize the scope of organizational and personal liability assumed and be agreeable to these terms. Agreements between third parties and the S/HMO and related contracts between the S/HMO corporate entity and participating providers must carefully spell out the risks assumed by each party.

Provider Incentives to Form S/HMOs

Given the nature of the risks inherent in capitation financing, the specification of provider incentives is of paramount importance for S/HMO growth potential. The primary incentives anticipated to induce providers to form S/HMOs are basically similar to the inducements for physician groups to develop prepaid group practices or HMOs. These incentives include: (1) savings incentives based on liberal, competitive capitation rates; (2) direct financial control over a sizable pool of resources and corresponding elimination of multiple third party billings and uneven, irregular cash flows; (3) elimination of the time and resources required to maintain multiple third party fee-for-service arrangements; (4) organizational stability and growth allowing for the solidification of client demand; and (5) the potential for innovation in the organization of the delivery system through the strategic use of alternative health and social services manpower.

Though all of these incentives are reasonably strong, a key incentive is the capitation sum negotiated and the corresponding arrangement for reallocation of cost savings below this sum. Currently, HMOs with Medicare risk sharing contracts negotiate reimbursement rates that are 95 percent of local average per capita costs for comparable services to persons over sixty-five. The savings potential for these HMOs increases the more they are able to lower costs below this 95 percent level. A similar approach to S/HMO rate setting is anticipated, though the process will be complicated by varying reimbursement formulas employed by major third party funders, alternative case mix and size assumptions, and the wide range of services to be included in the capitation rate. Whether or not 95 percent of per capita costs is an appropriate capitation rate will likely vary between locations. Savings formulas that include organizational savings plus savings passed on to enrollees are desirable as organizational incentives for S/HMO development.

During the initial stages of S/HMO development, rates would likely be negotiated frequently, perhaps even quarterly, to protect both the provider and the funding agencies. As S/HMO development stabilizes, rates would be negotiated yearly. In addition, target budgets covering a longer time period (for example, two to three years), which could project the health deterioration of the enrolled population, inflation, and other relevant factors, would provide a useful rate setting framework.

Working within an established capitation sum to achieve net savings poses a major challenge for the S/HMO provider entity. Unlike customary prepaid health plans, in which risk can be widely shared and actuarial analysis can be applied with a strong degree of confidence, the scope of services to be managed in the S/HMO and the corresponding estimates of utilization are more difficult to gauge. As a result, the S/HMO will need to screen service demands through tight controls over resource allocation.

Marketing Issues

A critical decision facing each S/HMO will be the question of enrolling the target population. Most Medicare enrollees in HMOs, for example, were members of an HMO prior to the time they were sixty-five. Neither HMOs nor other potential S/HMO providers have had significant experience in marketing a plan to the elderly.

One of the great challenges, therefore, facing providers interested in S/HMO formation is the development of a service package and capitation sum that will not only be attractive to public third party funders but also will be attractive to individuals and families. This service package must be sufficiently attractive for enrollees to forego their access to other local service providers and to pay out of pocket for the cost differential between the capitation established and limits of current public or private third party coverage. At a minimum, the S/HMO must convince members of the local target population that: (1) a guaranteed set of services is advantageous; (2) simplicity of access, flexibility and timeliness of response, and continuity of care are all improved through the S/HMO; (3) the services offered represent a better buy than current insurance programs; and (4) providers and institutions highly regarded in the community are participants in the S/HMO delivery network, thus minimizing the need to forego current provider relationships.

Developing a service package, a provider network capitation sum, and a marketing plan is a complex and time-consuming undertaking. Evidence exists that the elderly represent a group to whom marketing new service arrangements is difficult, although evidence also is available showing that the task is much easier if variations on an already existing organizational structure are being introduced rather than a completely new service delivery system (Lennox 1978). These are prime reasons why S/HMOs are anticipated to evolve from existing provider entities, rather than de novo.

Additional evidence shows that many elderly are without access to primary care providers (particularly in inner city and rural areas) and that the S/HMO might serve as a physician office substitute as well as a central point for accessing a wide range of supportive services. However, the possibility remains that needy populations beyond the immediate geographic radius of the S/HMO site might remain unserviced. In fact, this problem could be exacerbated if other community agencies drop current levels of service to the target population in deference to the S/HMO.

Enrollment in the S/HMO would be an ongoing process and would remain open subject to size and resource constraints and subject to maintaining the targeted case mix balance. Enrollees would have the option at particular points in time to withdraw if they so desired.

Since all S/HMOs will at some point need to engage in marketing their service package to potential enrollees not now in the direct user network, a specific marketing strategy specifying target populations by size, funding source, and functional condition will be necessary. A number of measures will be required of both the S/HMO and third party payors to assure that information about the S/HMO, its services, and provider network is readily available to potential enrollees. This information dissemination will need to be coupled with intensive community outreach.

The S/HMO will need to develop its own outreach staff to work closely with community agencies in an intensive, coordinated marketing effort. The extent of outreach and marketing for a given S/HMO will be tempered by the nature of the community and by the S/HMO's progress to that point in realizing its target enrollment. S/HMO services can also be marketed through private insurers, who are willing to offer riders on current health care policies to cover long-term-care services.

Quality-of-Care Issues

Given the range, intensity, and dollar magnitude of services an operational S/HMO must provide, consumers, regulators, and funders must all be assured that effective quality-control procedures are in place. In support of this effort, reimbursement incentives must be developed that make it difficult to engage either in creaming or failure to provide costly services when required. Several mechanisms could, if operating simultaneously, greatly temper the likelihood of such outcomes.

Peer review would likely be required in a systematic, organized manner, similar to the requirements for medical model HMOs. External program audits would reinforce and support internal peer review activities. Grievance procedures and the participation of users on advisory groups and on S/HMO boards of directors represent other potential quality input mechanisms. Boards may seek to increase the severity of case mix in order to reduce the likelihood of creaming. Furthermore, they may participate in the renegotiation of the capitation rate, which would include a thorough review of case mix, historical utilization, and cost experience.

Political Issues

Any major reorientation of a service delivery system would normally be expected to generate political tension, as entrenched interests anticipate competition from a new, unproven entity. The S/HMO is no exception, and a proposed S/HMO is likely to draw political fire from these sources: (1) consumers and planners, especially when the proposed provider has not demonstrated the capacity for such an undertaking; (2) community providers, especially those who may not be linked to the S/HMO; and (3) state- and local-government agencies, who must shoulder the burden for designing, monitoring, and regulating S/HMO development.

However, S/HMOs can be expected to be favored by those providers now operating one of the required program components, allied provider groups and community organizations, and sympathetic social agencies and consumers.

Conclusions

Certain conclusions can be drawn from performance data from potential S/HMO providers, as well as from our conceptual understanding of the S/HMO model, its potential variations, and anticipated developmental issues along with likely responses. The following sections discuss the anticipated system consequences of the S/HMO model and its anticipated benefits and outline policy recommendations that are designed to aid in the development of S/HMOs.

Anticipated System Consequences and Benefits
of the S/HMO Model

S/HMOs have been conceptually designed to correct certain deficiencies in the long-term-care service delivery system. Four major elements of the S/HMO model have been targeted to produce intended system consequences: (1) capitation through prepayment financing, (2) single provider to assume organizational responsibility, (3) comprehensive service benefit package, and (4) voluntary enrollment of participants. Table 8-5 lists the intended system consequences for each of these basic S/HMO elements.

Home health, personal care, and social services are likely to increase due to improved system controls in the S/HMO. Competition among existing agencies for contracts to provide these services may be high. New

Table 8-5
Generic S/HMO Elements and Intended System Consequences

Generic S/HMO Element	Intended System Consequences
Capitation Through Prepayment Financing	Greater emphasis on case management;
	Shift from inpatient services to ambulatory and home care services, when appropriate;
	Improved organizational planning and management systems and practices;
	Improved cash flow position;
	Direct provider control of reimbursements for all services rendered;
	Elimination of the burden of paper work for reimbursements for the managing-provider entity.
Single Provider to Assume Organizational Responsibility	Flexibility to innovate in creating an organized system of services;
	Direct accountability to users and public funders;
	Greater continuity of care and integration of diverse service elements.
Comprehensive Service Benefit Package	Guaranteed coverage through one source for comprehensive health care and related personal support needs;
	Greater simplicity of the long-term-care system;
	Potential of wider service benefits at no additional consumer or public third-party costs.
Voluntary Enrollment of Participants	Guarantee of availability of needed services;
	Community prevention and education efforts as part of S/HMO marketing;
	Consumer participation in S/HMO decision making.

organizations might be induced into the marketplace or growth of existing agencies could fill identified gaps. Additional manpower, especially chore workers, homemakers, home health aides, and visiting nurses, may be required over time. Some might be directly added to the core staff, while others might be contracted to community agencies. The growth of specialized health personnel to staff acute-care hospitals and nursing homes might, in time, be moderately arrested through the presence of the S/HMO. The strength of this effect would depend on the age and case mix characteristics of the particular target population, as well as on other related factors.

Redistribution of dollars toward home care and personal support services is anticipated. In time, this redistribution might be of considerable magnitude. Eventually, overall per capita costs are expected to be comparable or lower than for similar populations served through individual fee-for-service providers. Although initial start-up costs will be high due to organizational development, marketing and outreach efforts, and the introduction of required administrative support mechanisms over a period of time, net systems savings are anticipated.

Judging the distribution of dollars from potential federal and state sources is difficult, since distribution will depend upon the target population, resource constraints, and program priorities. Public funding is best viewed as an investment from which gains are captured after a build-up period. More federal dollars are likely at program initiation with savings emerging after a phase-in period. Additional state dollars may also be required, depending on the percent of Medicaid buy-ins and available Title XX buy-in funds. Maximization of federal funds and a shift of state funds from institutional to home-based services are anticipated. However, the bottom line effect after the build-up period should be more containable and controllable public expenditures, despite investment in the new delivery form.

The management tools, assessment and quality-control instruments, and financial controls developed and operated by the S/HMO provider would have direct and important system control consequences. Of particular importance for the S/HMO will be the successful development of management information systems, instruments for assessment and diagnosis, provider quality-control assessment tools, paper-flow management techniques including a viable design for patient records flow, reimbursement and related case flow systems, and effective means of interagency communications and record keeping. Furthermore, the services and resource controls at the disposal of the S/HMO will provide it with considerable system development influence. For example, its role in brokering services will likely foster the growth of particular community-based services such as homemaker and chore services.

A strong shift toward centralized patient management is also anticipated through the S/HMO. System entry, patient assessment, certification, and case management including referral, advocacy, and follow-up are the anticipated control functions of the S/HMO. Of the various long-term-care reforms currently under consideration, the S/HMO offers the strongest possibility of centralized controls over patient management, and hence may offer the greatest potential for efficiency and cost savings.

For consumers, greater freedom of choice and an increased role in decision making is anticipated under an S/HMO model. The S/HMO staff team would be generally expected to work with clients and their families in designing and implementing a service package and risk management strategy most desirable in light of the client's prevailing condition at enrollment.

Underlying all these anticipated changes is the assumption that S/HMOs will produce substitution of home- and community-based services for institutional or other health-focused care, a greater degree of continuity of care, and stronger agency commitments to provide services that will maintain functional stability and retard deterioration (Winn and McCaffree 1978).

Policy Recommendations

A number of constraints to S/HMO development have been suggested in this chapter, including administrative complexity, current provider capacity, political opposition of selected provider groups, and ability to enroll the target population. On the more positive side, several studies were cited illustrating cost and organizational effectiveness of HMOs and PCOs in providing a comprehensive range of services to elderly target populations. Interest has been expressed by several of these organizations in moving toward a capitated arrangement. S/HMOs through ORDS (Office of Research, Demonstrations, and Statistics) and HCFA demonstration monies are now in development in a few sites (see appendix 8A) and have become one of the most interesting new concepts to be developed through the National Long-Term-Care Demonstration Project. These sites should help answer a fundamental question for government policymakers: To what extent should public support catalyze S/HMO development and, if such development is warranted, how can S/HMOs best be implemented?

On balance, sufficient positive evidence exists for long-term-care capitation to warrant incremental evolution of S/HMOs. The number of provider organizations immediately able to mount an S/HMO trial development effort is probably no more than one to two dozen. The costs of an effort of this magnitude can likely be absorbed through the level of demonstration monies now available to HCFA, ORDS, OHMOS (Office of Health Maintenance Organizations) and the Public Health Service during the next few fiscal years. But if the trials prove successful, then dozens of other established provider groups that already exist could form the core of a nationwide S/HMO network.

The advantage of this approach is that the S/HMO network can start without a major new infusion of funds and without any new legislative mandate or initiative. A combination of these sources, beginning with demonstration projects, might facilitate the development of five to ten S/HMOs during the next two years. After sufficient time for field evaluation and research, a decision about more intensified follow-up efforts can be more judiciously made. The initial effort might reach a small percentage of the total elderly population now at risk of institutionalization, especially those persons currently receiving minimal home care support services. The initial S/HMO development efforts, described in appendix 8A, will serve as pilot tests for a broader implementation strategy that could commence during FY 1981.

Note

1. The key concepts of an S/HMO-insurance, social service benefits, and capitation have been proposed by Morris since 1975. See *Annual Report*, Levinson Policy Institute, Brandeis University, Waltham, Mass., September 1975; D. Bergsma and A. Pulver, eds., "Alternative Forms of Care for the Disabled: Developing Community Services," *Developmental Disabilities*, New York: Allen Liss, 1976; "Per Capita Assessment: A Local Approach to Public Home Care Insurance," Levinson Policy Institute, Brandeis University, Waltham, Mass., September 1975; "The Personal Care Organization: An Approach to Long-Term Care Delivery," Select Committee on Aging, Subcommittee on Health Maintenance and Long-Term Care Testimony, June 11, 1975, Washington, D.C.

Appendix 8A
Field Testing of the
S/HMO: Activities to Date

During the past year, a staff team based at the University Health Policy Consortium conducted initial field explorations at several sites to test the viability of the S/HMO concept in the eyes of a range of local providers. The providers contacted included an acute-care hospital that is part of a group of hospitals and nursing homes; two community-care organizations; three federally qualified HMOs; and two physician group practices, one tied to a network of inner-city-neighborhood health centers. Each of these entities directly provides a broad range of health and social services to a sizable elderly population (2,500-10,000). Five states were represented, inclusive of the east coast, west coast, and midwest.

As part of the initial test of the viability of the S/HMO concept, each interested provider was asked to identify in a preliminary fashion the following:

Size and scope of the proposed target population and case-mix controls;

Services benefits now provided, by whom, and benefits proposed under an S/HMO model including proposed service deliverers;

Profile of current service utilizations and aggregate costs among the proposed target population;

Marketing/enrollment strategy and targets;

Proposed corporate organization and the specific relationships among selected staff;

The current component parts of the service-delivery system and proposed new contractual arrangements under an operating S/HMO;

Case management system currently utilized and how this function might be adjusted in the S/HMO;

Peer review and related quality-control mechanisms in place and refinements required in an S/HMO mode;

Waivers that would be required to operate the S/HMO.

The findings of these initial field analyses provided sufficiently strong evidence of feasibility to warrant further development and testing of the S/HMO. The cross section of providers studied demonstrates strong case management, information, referral, and growth capacities, as well as the ability to manage a wide variety of essential long-term-care services utilizing a number of institutional service substitutes. In addition, most were experienced in public third party contracting and in securing supporting program waivers. The providers as a group were uniformly interested in fully testing an operational S/HMO model.

As a result of these initial findings, University Health Policy Consortium staff submitted administration grant application to the Health Care Financing Administration for resources to design, support, and oversee a three-year field test of the S/HMO in at least three alternative agency settings. This grant has been funded and this effort will continue through the 1983 fiscal year. Site selection will be made in the Winter/Spring of 1981. Simultaneously, an external evaluator will be selected.

References

Bernier, E., and Quinn, J. 1980. "Triage: An Alternative Care System for the Elderly, 1974-1979." Rockville, Md.: HEW.

Donabedian, A. 1969. "An Evaluation of Prepaid Group Practice." *Inquiry* 6 (3):3-27.

Eggert, G.M., et al. 1978. *Monroe County Long-Term Care Demonstration Project: Initial Six Month Progress Report* Rochester, N.Y.

Gaus, C.; Cooper, B.; and Hirschman, C. 1976. "Contrasts in HMO and Fee-For-Service Performance." *Social Security Bulletin* 39 (5):3-19.

Germane, Pearl; Skinner, Elizabeth; and Shapiro, Sam. 1976. "Ambulatory Care for Chronic Conditions in an Inner City Elderly Population." *American Journal of Public Health* 66 (7):660-666.

Hurtado, A., et al. 1972. "Utilization and Costs of a Home Care and Extended Services in a Prepaid Group Practice." *Medical Care* 10 (1): 8-16.

Jones, E.; Densen, P.; Altman, I.; Shapiro, S.; and West, H. 1974. "HIP Incentive Reimbursement Experiment: Utilization and Costs of Medical Care, 1969 and 1970." *Social Security Bulletin* 37 (12):3-34.

Lennox, K. 1978. *HMOs as an Alternative Mode of Care for the Elderly.* Washington, D.C.: Urban Institute.

Luft, H.S. 1978. "How Do Health Maintenance Organizations Achieve Their 'Savings'?" *New England Journal of Medicine* 298:1336-1343.

Meltzer, J., and Joe, T. 1979. *Policies and Strategies for Long-Term Care.* San Francisco: Health Policy Program, School of Medicine, University of California.

Pearson, David C. 1975. "Elements of Progressive Patient Care in the Yale Health Plan." *Public Health Reports* 29 (2):119-125.

Pollak, W. 1978. *Expanding Health Benefits for the Elderly: Long-Term Care*, Vol. I. Washington, D.C.: The Urban Institute.

Roemer, M. 1978. Testimony before the Subcommittee on Health and Long-Term Care on HMOs and the Elderly. Washington, D.C., May.

Social Security Administration, Office of Research and Statistics. 1978. *Census of Medicare Contracted HMOs*. Washington, D.C.

Weil, P. 1976. "Comparative Costs to the Medicare Program of Seven Prepaid Group Practice Plans." *Milbank Fund Quarterly* (Summer):339-365.

Winn, S., and McCaffree, K. 1978. *Issues in the Development of a Prepaid System of Long-Term Care Services*. Seattle: Batelle Research.

A Systems Approach
to Long-Term Care

James J. Callahan, Jr.

Long-term care involves a confusingly heterogeneous population to be
served and a confusing array of more-or-less independent provider and
financing organizations that are only weakly integrated. An understanding
of this complex, very loosely articulated system is necessary for a proper
evaluation of any option for long-term-care reform for one reason—the
system does function after a fashion in meeting the needs of several million
citizens. Any major option, if adopted, would impose significant changes
on the way that system works. Understanding the functions and processes
of the system is important if it is to serve people better. Also important,
however, is estimating the extent to which any option may disrupt, rather
than improve, the functioning of the system. Therefore, elaborating on the
nature of this system as a context for considering specific financing and
organizational reforms is worthwhile.

A Systems Approach

Sayles and Chandler (1971), in their study of the NASA program, describe
the complex processes and interactions necessary to accomplish large-scale
public objectives in modern society. They note two significant characteristics of these large-scale efforts that have relevance to solving the problem
of long-term care.

> First, all these objectives imply the collaboration of a relatively large
> number of organizations, and it would appear that these will be a mixture
> of public and private institutions. . . . Many new developments depend
> upon close, collaborative, and integrated activities that crisscross organiza-
> tional boundaries and the dividing line between public and private
> sectors. . . . A second element common to many large programs is uncer-
> tain technology. [Sayles and Chandler 1971, pp. 2-3]

These interdependencies and uncertainties are reflected in the growing
emphasis on systems: systems management, urban systems, the systems approach, and so on.

The problems most frequently associated with long-term care are
developed in chapter 2. Solving these problems certainly can be considered

as a large-scale public objective of the type identified by Sayles and Chandler (1971). Anyone familiar with the field is aware of the scope and the complexity of the public/private mixture and the uncertainties of management. A systems approach may prove useful as a means to understand better the problems of long-term care.

A first step in applying systems thinking is to identify the objective that reflects what the system is supposed to do. The requirements necessary to reach an objective are the components and resources of the system. The system operates within an environment with exchange across its boundaries. Within the system, allocative processes occur that distribute roles, resources, and responsibilities. Integrative processes are also at work that mesh various activities toward the system objective. In order to continue, the system must maintain some type of equilibrium to achieve objectives. Because of this equilibrium requirement, note that some activities are incompatible with a particular array of functions. It, therefore, may not be possible to optimize both cost control and provider discretion. Combining systemwide planning and service delivery in one agency may turn out to be undesirable. Only by an examination of system functions and processes can answers to these questions be developed.

One aspect of systems theory that will not be discussed to any degree is the concept of the system environment. The environment essentially represents the givens within which the system operates and upon which the system has little influence, although we recognize that systems affect their environments. In one sense, the population that becomes the input to the system is part of the environment. The financial resources of the society as well as attitudes toward their use (for example, the Proposition-13 mentality) would be part of the environment.

Many suggestions are offered about what to do with the long-term-care system. Some of these suggestions are aimed at improving attainment of system objectives—for example, actions that will increase a person's degree of independence. This class of suggestions could be termed *system-outcome oriented*. On the other hand, proposals to reduce costs of long-term care may or may not improve outcomes but are a necessary system response to environmental pressures. These responses would be considered *system-adaptation responses*. The distinction between these two responses as decisions are made about the long-term-care system will be important.

Conceptual Framework

The conceptual framework proposed is based upon some basic principles of systems theory. No single systems theory is being used, but relevant concepts have been selected from various authors: Sayles and Chandler (1971), Churchman (1968), and Parsons and Shills (1962).

The central core of the population to be affected is made up of individuals who are identified as functionally dependent—that is, needing some attention and care from another adult over long, ill-defined periods of time. Around this core spreads a larger population of persons with variable disabilities and dependencies who, with their families, make up the larger pool of potential users. The state of functional dependence is affected by several factors, the more significant being: medical treatability, physical-rehabilitation potential, extent of informal supports available (family or friends), extent of agency supports available, and income. The make-up of this pool is constantly shifting as individuals deteriorate or improve in their capacities, as population cohorts age, and as medical science keeps disabled younger people alive for longer periods of time. Thus, the target population is characterized by change.

Figure 9-1 shows the long-term-care system at its most general level of conception. The input is a patient described in terms of variables: age, sex, race, marital status, living arrangement, vision, hearing, communication abilities, activities of daily living, mobility, adaptive tasks, disruptive behavior, orientation/memory impairment, and disturbance of mood.

These variables were selected from the U.S. National Committee on Vital and Health Statistics (1979). The document represents about two years of work of a technical-consultant panel. The data set defines a central core of data about a given dimension of health and health services needed on a routine basis by the majority of users. The document also includes standardized definitions, measurements, and classifications. Although our ability to actually measure and assess various states is limited, this document calls attention to the important variables.

The box in the center of the figure represents the long-term-care system and will be filled in at increased levels of detail in later diagrams.

The outputs on the right-hand side represents the objective(s) of the system as noted in the literature.

1. Maximum functional independence
   a. Rehabilitation
   b. Maintenance
2. Humane care
   a. Least-restrictive environment
   b. Death with dignity
3. Prolong longevity
4. Prevent avoidable medical/social problems

Obviously, the objectives to be sought would vary by the needs of the per-

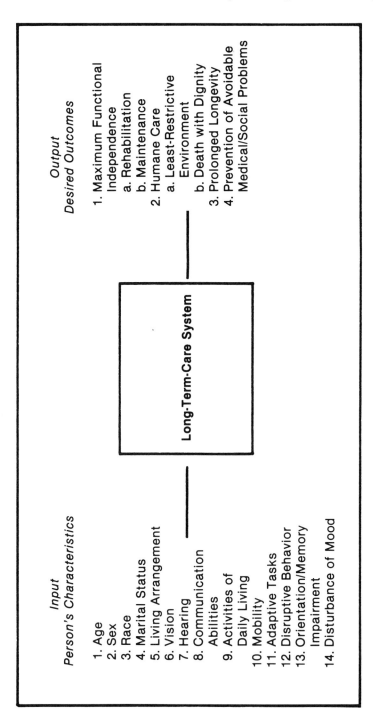

Figure 9-1. Long-Term-Care System Input-Output Overview

Source: U.S. National Committee on Vital and Health Statistics, National Center for Health Statistics, Public Health Service, DHEW. *Long-Term Health Care: Minimum Data Set.* (Washington, D.C. May 1979).

son who enters the system. An accident victim might be rehabilitated. An elderly person at home might be helped to maintain functional independence. A seriously disabled adult may not be able to achieve more than humane care, while a long-term cancer victim may die in a dignified manner. There may be other objectives of the long-term-care system, and there may not be agreement on the objectives selected. However, a clear understanding of the objectives will be important before one begins to wrestle with the construction of a system or organization for long-term care.

Figure 9-2 lays out the functions of the long-term-care system. These functions are the categories of activities that the system must perform if the objectives are to be obtained. The functions set down in figure 9-2 were derived from a review of significant literature in the field (see appendix A). Long-term-care activities identified by the various authors were recorded and categorized under functional headings. The intent was to find a place for all the activities mentioned. Some activities were mentioned more frequently than others, but no attempt was made to weight the importance of functions by the number of mentions. The intent, rather, was to be comprehensive. Some of these functions may not be necessary. Possibly, perhaps probably, additional functions are not described. The justification for this approach is that these functions are what the experts say are the important considerations. In actually applying the framework additional functions could be discovered.

The system functions are arranged under three headings: systems management, operational management, and patient management. These levels are intended to reflect differences in management scope, level, and responsibility.

Figures 9-3, 9-4, and 9-5 attempt to identify some of the components (agencies and organizations) that perform the system functions. Where possible, federal, state, and local entities have been identified. This listing is intended to be suggestive of types of organizations, not an exhaustive list of every agency in the field. The listing, however, does give a picture of the number and types of actors involved in long-term care. These figures are revealing in that it shows that federal-government involvement is almost exclusively at the systems-management level. Local involvement is greatest at the patient-management level. The state role is not clear, but it does have some function at all three levels. A change in role at one level of government (for example, the federal) would significantly affect the other levels.

The following sections describe briefly each function and list the major organizational components of each. No attempt is made to analyze the relationships among the components of a particular function or to analyze the relationships among the total system components. Such analyses would be a useful contribution to understanding long-term care but is beyond the scope of this work.

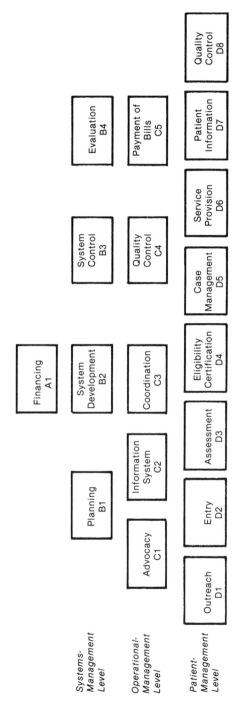

Figure 9-2. Long-Term-Care-System Array of Functions

Systems Management Functions

Provision of Financial Resources. The provision of financial resources is a systems-management function that is basic to all the other functions. From figure 9-2, obviously all the functions from planning to service delivery to advocacy require funding. From where will the resources be acquired? What mechanisms exist or will exist to allocate these funds? Will the amount of resources increase or decrease? How well developed are the financing resources of various types of services? From where will financing come to underwrite system-development activities? Financing will be discussed in more detail later. The main point here is that all system activities need to be financed, not just patient services, and the sources of financing are varied.

Components: HCFA (Titles XVIII, XIX)
OHDS (Title XX)
AoA (Title III)
VA, HUD
State Medicaid Agency
State Title XX Agency
State Mental Health
County Institutions
Local Matching Funds

Planning. Planning is an important function in the long-term-care system. The need was explicitly noted by various authors. Specific statements included "comprehensive planning," "identification of disabled and elder population," "cataloging of resources." Planning in the long-term-care system would involve all the activities usually associated with planning and would face many of the usual constraints, if not more. Very little, however, has been written on how this planning would take place, and this function will require detailed expansion.

Components: HCFA (Titles XVIII, XIX)
OHDS (Title XX)
AoA (Title III)
State HSA
State DoN
AAA
State A95
State Title XX
Regional HSA
Local Planning Councils

System Development. The system-development function is conceived as "maintaining a sufficient supply of services and facilities" and/or "development of resources." System development is analytically distinct from the planning function in that it would include capital funding, establishment of new organizations, mergers, manpower development, and other related activities.

Components: HCFA (Titles XVIII, XIX)
OHDS (Title XX)
State Health Department

System Control. System control refers to the management of the levers that can influence the behavior of components of the system. These levers include regulation, legal authority, control of funding allocations, certificate of need, certification of providers, sign-off and review, market interactions, rate setting, and veto power. Controls may be decentralized and of a market nature or highly centralized and regulated. The function of control on a centralized basis is seen as very important by some policymakers in long-term care as the only way to achieve desired outcomes.

Components: HCFA (Titles VII, XIX)
OHDS (Title XX)
AoA (Title III)
State Title XX
State Rate Setting
State Health Department

Evaluation. Evaluation is concerned with how the overall system functions. It is analytically distinct from quality control, which is concerned with a particular individual. Quality control, for example, would be concerned about a particular day-care center's performance according to some standard. (Although quality control might be considered part of the operations phase of evaluation, we consider it useful to treat them separately.) Evaluation, on the other hand, would examine the extent to which day care as a service is a necessary component of the long-term-care system. Evaluative criteria for long-term care frequently mentioned include:

Cost effectiveness of various modalities of long-term care,

Coordination of services,

Comprehensiveness of services,

Efficient operation of programs.

These items may be considered internal evaluative criteria for the operation of the system. The outcomes listed in figure 9-1 (independence, humaneness) represent the output evaluation criteria of the system. The evaluative function is concerned with measuring system performance around both sets of criteria. This function, however, was not frequently described in the literature.

Components: HCFA (Titles XVIII, XIX)
             OHDS (Title XX)
             NIA

Operational Management Functions

Advocacy. Advocacy refers to activity around a particular individual to ensure receipt of entitlements and benefits. It would include "path finding," legal representation, patient rights (for example, client participation, privacy), reasonable travel distance to service, and so on. Advocacy may also be on a system basis to produce changes in law, policy, and regulations.

Components: AAA
             Developmental Disabilities
             Legal Services Agency
             Special Population Interest Groups
             (for example, Handicapped)

Management-Information System. This system includes the organization and processing of data among the entities comprising the service-delivery system.

Components: Medicare Intermediaries
             State Title XX Agency
             Local Consortia

Coordination. This element refers to the coordination of the available community resources to reduce fragmentation and improve efficient use of resources. Coordination is further refined to include integration of services and implementation structures and networks. The focus here is around community-level coordination, not case coordination. It would include joint funding and budgeting, joint planning, development of common operating policies, and similar mechanisms.

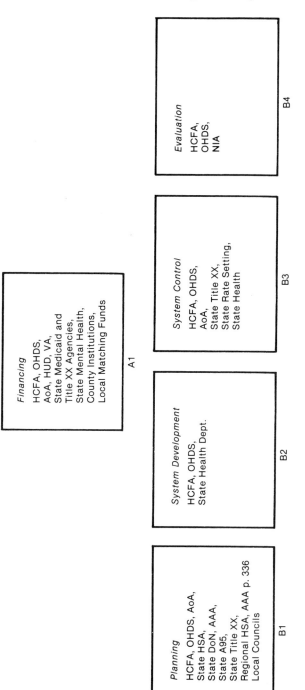

Figure 9-3. Long-Term-Care-System Systems-Management Components

Components: Title XX Agency
                AAA
                HSA

Quality Control. Quality control includes those activities referred to as performance monitoring, quality assurance, monitoring of services, and the like. At this level, it concerns quality control around service entities, not individuals.

Components: PSRO
                State Health Department
                Local Health Department
                Professional Societies
                Advocacy Groups

Payment of Bills. Bill payment was not mentioned in the literature, but it is a very important function. It is distinct from the general category of financing and has to do with cash flow and getting money to providers for services delivered.

Components: Medicare Intermediaries (HCFA)
                Title XIX Agency
                Title XX Agency
                Title III (COAA) Agency
                Users

Patient-Management Functions

Outreach. This function includes activities designed to publicize a service, to identify and contact potential users, and to get clients to the service (for example, transportation).

Components: AAA
                Senior Centers
                Ad hoc Enrollment Program (for example, SSI)
                Poverty Agencies

Entry. Entry is seen as an important consideration. All authors agree that entry should be at the community level. The entry point should be such that it facilitates access to the system. Control of entry into the system is seen by some professionals to be the key to managing the system, particularly as it affects institutional care.

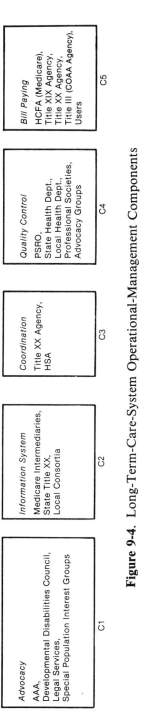

Figure 9-4. Long-Term-Care-System Operational-Management Components

An open system is one in which a person need not formally enter the system through a designated point to obtain a service or set of services. The person may choose to obtain the services on his own directly from a provider, or go through the designated long-term-care entry point. A closed system would be one in which all potential service users would have to go through a mandated entry point(s). There could be single or multiple points in a community, and they could be designated for all groups or particular groups (for example, elderly, disabled, children). Criteria need to be developed for selecting among these possibilities.

Components: Hospitals
Nursing Homes
HHA
Homemaker Agencies
Title XX Agency or Contractor
Public Health Departments
Special Projects (for example, Triage)
AAA

Individual Assessment of Need. The various authors all agree highly that the system must perform an individual needs assessment. This is indeed an important function of the system. How it gets done, by whom, with what patient participation, and with what assessment tool are, among others, very important considerations.

Components: Hospitals
Nursing Homes
HHA
Homemaker Agencies
Title XX Agency or Contractor
Public Health Departments
Special Projects (for example, Triage)
AAA

Eligibility/Certification Function. This function is related to the needs assessment but is different in that it confers a particular entitlement on an individual. It may include the following:

Conferring eligibility for the services of the entire care plan;

Designating a level of care and certifying an individual for reimbursement purposes;

Arranging a care plan based on an individual's current eligibility under multiple programs (for example, Medicare, Veteran's Administration, and so on);

No entitlements—eligibility based on availability of funds.

Components: HCFA (Medicare, Medicaid)
             State Title XIX Agency
             State Title XX Agency
             Special Projects

Case Management. Case management is a frequently mentioned essential function of the long-term-care system. Its various functions are:

Collaborating arrangements to assure continuity of service regardless of the auspice of the provider,

Making necessary care arrangements,

Referring and coordinating appropriate service,

Arranging for covered items and services,

Maintaining a continuous relationship with the individual,

Being a broker by matching individual needs and resources,

Insuring delivery of services.

While this function is described in various ways, it is based on the fact that long-term-care individuals usually have more than one need and must have contact with more than one provider. It reflects also the fact that these needs are chronic and continuous, rather than random and episodic; hence, the need for case management over time.

Components: Title XX Agency or Providers
             AAA
             Special Projects
             Developmental Disabilities Agency

Service Provision. Service provision is the major function of the long-term-care system. The following listing shows the range of services and providers currently used by long-term-care individuals.

Patient-Information System. This refers to particular patient-based record systems.

Component: All Providers
            Family
            Case-Management Agency

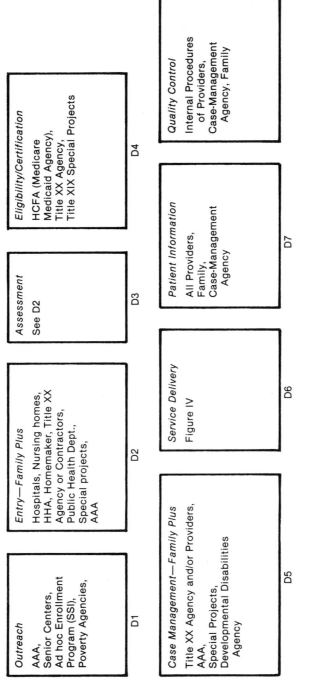

Figure 9-5. Long-Term-Care-System Patient-Management Components

Quality Control. Quality control includes activities to insure that a particular organization is performing up to some standard and/or that a particular client has received a particular service meeting a designated standard.

Components: Licensing/Certification Bodies
Case Management Agency
Provider
PSRO

Table 9-1
Long-Term-Care Services and Provider Agencies

Services	*Providers*
Chore	General hospital
Home health	Specialty hospital
Transportation	Nursing home
	Residential facility
Social services	Hospice
Personal care (ADL)	Mental-health center
Nursing	Home-health center
Legal assistance	Homemaker agency
Nutritionist/dietitian	Day hospital
Telephone reassurance	Day-care center
	Sheltered workshop
MD-Do Services	Hospital emergency rooms
Other medical (dentists, optometrists)	Neighborhood health center
Counseling	Multipurpose senior centers
Information and referral	HMO
	Public social-service agency
Physical therapy	Public-health agency
Occupational therapy	Individual practitioners
	Voluntary social-service agency
Nursing home	Vocational rehabilitation agency
Residential care	Employment agency
	Adult activity centers for handicapped
Day care	Library
Friendly visiting	Recreation agencies
Recreation	Public housing authority
Protective service	Public/private transportation
Speech and hearing	companies
Assessment service	Halfway house
Foster care	Foster home
Meals-on-wheels	Church/synagogue
Congregate meals	Community long-term-care center
Case management	Outreach
Mental health	Sitting service
Job assistance	Escort service
Sheltered employment	Laundry service
Emergency care	Placement service
Respite care	Special support groups
Preretirement counseling	Hospice care
Equipment loan	Night/day partial hospital or
Shopping assistance	residential care
Congregate housing	Family members
Day health care	

Conclusion

The description of system functions and components, while useful, does not tell us how the system actually works. Nor does it tell us what the various outcomes of any reform might be. It does, however, help us in knowing where to look for results and in developing hypotheses. It is useful also in identifying what specific functions and components are addressed by particular options and which functions are excluded.

This analysis does point up the need for theory development in long-term care. Without some explanatory framework it will be impossible to understand the workings of so many components' performing so many functions around so many individual problems and needs. Social-policy formulation in the absence of theory may offer some politically attractive solutions in the short run but will not establish a firm base for meeting the needs of our handicapped and disabled citizens.

References

Churchman, C.W. 1968. *The Systems Approach*. New York: Delacorte Press.

Parsons, T., and Shills, E.A., eds. 1962. *Toward a General Theory of Action*. New York: Harper Torch Books.

Sayles, L.R., and Chandler, M.K., 1971. *Managing Large Systems: Organizations for the Future* New York: Harper & Row.

U.S. National Committee on Vital and Health Statistics, National Center for Health Statistics, Public Health Service, DHEW. 1979. *Long-Term Health Care: Minimum Data Set*. Washington, D.C., May.

Appendix A:
Previous Analyses of
Major Reform Options
for Long-Term Care

Paul Youket

The purpose of this appendix is to present a synthesis of the analyses of major reform option for long-term care that have been done previously. Seven former analyses are identified: Congressional Budget Office (CBO)(1977), Correia (1976), Joe and Meltzer (1976), Pollak (1974), and U.S. Department of Health, Education, and Welfare (HEW) (1974, 1976, 1978).

Rather than describe each paper separately, their contributions are discussed according to the financing or organizational characteristics of the options analyzed. The varying level of discussion corresponds to the depth of treatment provided by the authors. The options are organized into groupings similar to those presented in this volume.

The financing options include: cash payment, vouchers/disability allowance, national health insurance, federal/state matching programs (open-ended and close-ended), and mixed financing system (specialization program funding for long-term care setting, need or cost). The organization options include the use of local long-term care agencies.

Cash Payments

This option is considered by Pollak (1974) and Correia (1976). According to Pollak, cash grants would be given to eligible clients in proportion to their assessed level of need. Clients would then be free to purchase whatever services from whatever providers they wished. (Correia does not define this option.)

Correia and Pollak agree that such a program would maximize the flexibility of recipients in meeting their long-term-care needs and in matching services to their particular circumstances but that the cost of such a program would be very high. Pollak considers high cost to be a problem shared by all of the options he reviews, while Correia thinks that such a program would be potentially the most costly of all because very high payments would have to be made for recipients to be able to purchase institutional care.

Pollak and Correia disagree explicitly about the administrative difficulty and complexity of this option. Pollak, on the one hand, believes that a cash-payment program would present fewer administrative complexities than a vendor-payment program. Correia, on the other hand, states that a cash-payment program would be the most difficult system to administer because persons would have a strong incentive to exaggerate their disabilities. He concludes that such an approach is unworkable because of its high cost and its administrative difficulties.

Pollak (1974) makes a number of other points about this option. He considers cash payments to be only a particular form of program benefits and "a way of organizing service delivery which is compatible with several financing, federal/state, and other choices" (p. 45). Deductibles and co-insurance could be translated into differential cash grants to persons with similar needs for care but with different incomes. However, coinsurance "does not serve a rationing function with cash grants since the level of payment is determined administratively rather than by client behavior or influenced by cost sharing" (p. 46). In cases in which the level of demand is very small in particular areas, the market may not respond with a sufficient supply of desired services, so that "an organizational form which more directly regulates or manages supply may be required" (p. 23). Many individuals with long-term-care needs may be incapable of making competent selections of services and providers in the market. Economic and political pressure may also dictate the provision of particular services to meet specific identified needs created by impairments. "Politicians . . . may be reluctant to support a cash program which permits neglect of those problems—even if the program is in some sense better for the persons to whom it is directed" (p. 24). The level of cash grants given to clients should be different for institutional care than for home care and clients should be required to select one or the other type of care before the amount of their cash grant is determined. If the levels of the grants were the same for all settings, then the program would unnecessarily incur costs above the minimum level needed to meet needs for care in the least costly setting. If the primary objective of cash grants, however, is to provide "flexibility in fitting services to [clients'] own life styles," then they might only be appropriate for home care, since such variation is not likely to exist for institutional care (p. 46). The amount of the grant given to a recipient may also have to be a function of the recipient's family status. A cash-grant program would offer the same improvements over present programs for financing long-term care as a special insurance program would if the schedules of the two programs were similar.

Vouchers

Only Pollak (1974) considers vouchers for long-term care. He defines such vouchers as "dollar-valued rights" for the purchase of "a restricted set of care services or a set thought broadly appropriate to the needs of the particular individual" (pp. 19-20). He specifies two types of vouchers: vendor payments that are open-ended vouchers and voucher payments that are closed-ended vouchers whose value equals the costs of meeting an individual's assessed needs for care less any applicable deductibles and coinsurance.

Pollak considers vouchers to be only a form of program benefits and a way of organizing the supply of services. He says that although open-ended vouchers are logically identical to vendor payments, they are different administratively. "Since at least some included services may be close substitutes for normally purchased goods and services," some mechanisms, such as coinsurance deductibles and copayments, "will . . . be required to limit requests for open-ended vouchers in order to contain program costs directly and to minimize the inflationary impact of voucher-financed purchases on service prices" (p. 20). Other mechanisms that more directly control service prices may also be necessary for open-ended vouchers. Consumer choice would determine service mix, prices, and costs, and suppliers would be accountable for their services to consumers in the market. Consumers would be more likely to "police service prices" with (close-ended) voucher payments, so that "direct regulation of prices is less likely to be required . . . " (p. 22). The use of vouchers may be politically and economically more advantageous than the use of cash payments and would involve "minimum sacrifice" of the advantages of a cash approach (p. 24). Their use would also "assure" and "advertise the existence of" demand for the desired set of services and "would thereby stimulate the production of services . . . which would not otherwise be available" (p. 25). As with cash payments, however, not all individuals with needs for long-term care may be capable of making effective consumer choices in the market. A "public-coordinator/private-supply mode" might be required for those who cannot (p. 25).[1]

Long-Term Care Benefits Covered under National Health Insurance

This option is discussed briefly by Joe and Meltzer (1976) and Pollak (1974). Joe and Meltzer conclude that long-term care should not be part of a national health insurance program unless no alternative program is available, because all proposals consider only institutional long-term care, because it would maintain arbitrary classifications of institutions and the arbitrary division between health and nonhealth long-term-care services, and because including nonmedical services under national health insurance would be extremely expensive and would tend to confine long-term care to a medical model. Pollak states only that cost sharing for institutional long-term care under national health insurance should be higher than for acute care and that, if community long-term care is covered under such a program, formal care may be substituted for informal care, and more controls on utilization would be needed because there is a greater potential for overuse.

Separate Social Insurance Program

The insurance option has been looked at by the CBO (1977), Correia (1976), HEW (1974), and Pollak (1974). This would be a federally administered, individual-entitlement program. Federal financing would be open-ended and drawn from general revenues. There would be no premium payments or enrollment, but patient cost sharing would be required. State participation could be made either mandatory or optional. Eligibility and benefits would be federally defined. SNF and ICF care would be fully covered, but former analyses differ on the extent of coverage of noninstitutional care. Similarly, the elderly and the disabled would be fully covered, but coverage of other populations is not clear. The nonpoor would be covered through the use of income-related, cost-sharing schedules. Under two of the analyses (CBO 1977; HEW 1974), entitlement to services would be based on the existence of a medical condition or disability. Certification would be done by providers, by so-called community disability-certification centers, or by community long-term-care centers. Payments to providers would be made through state fiscal intermediaries or through community long-term-care centers.

Such a program would provide nationally uniform and more-equitable coverage of populations and benefits. A better balance would be formed between institutional care and noninstitutional care due to more equal coverage. The costs of such a program are difficult to predict but are likely to be very high. Although cost sharing and other mechanisms would help, control over the utilization of services would be difficult, especially for noninstitutional services. The quality of institutional care would be improved through higher federal rates of reimbursement and through better federal enforcement of standards. Federal regulation and intervention are likely to be extensive and may not be adequately responsive to local circumstances.

Federal/State Matching Program with Open-Ended Federal Funding

This type of option is considered principally by HEW (1974) and, to a limited degree, by Pollak (1974). According to HEW (1974), this would be an optional program administered by the states under federal guidelines and regulations and financed through open-ended, federal/state matching grants "based on state per capita income and state-determined need" (p. 32). The federal government would specify minimum requirements, but the states would determine the specific characteristics of their own programs. Eligibility would be based on medical disability, income, and asset criteria; the nonpoor would be covered through the use of cost sharing schedules. Both institutional and noninstitutional, and both health and social services, would be covered, although some would be optional.

According to HEW (1974), such a program would make "a common benefit package of health and health-related services available to low income persons through one centralized state administered program" (p. 34). States would be able to merge such a program with Title XX, if the matching grant formulas for both programs were the same. Better coverage of noninstitutional services would expand the range of possible care settings and allow more persons to remain in residential settings. "Interstate variations would be minimal for mandated benefits, but could be considerable where states determine eligibility, cost sharing and standards for providers" (p. 35). Since states would be totally responsible for provider certification under this program, two separate sets of providers could develop, one certified under more strict federal requirements for national health insurance, and the other certified under less strict state standards under this program. Although states would have more direct control over the utilization of services under this program, such control would still be difficult.

Both HEW (1974) and Pollak consider such an option to be very similar to the insurance option, the main difference being that, under the latter, the program would be federally administered, while under the former, it would be state administered. Consequently, Pollak limits his observations on this option to the need for management-information systems, client-information and referral systems, and experimental data to make cost projections.

Grants to States with Closed-Ended Federal Funding

All of the previous analyses, except Joe and Meltzer's (1976), address this option. Under this option, states would receive closed-ended formula grants from the federal government. A full range of long-term-care services would be covered—institutional and noninstitutional, health and social. States would have wide discretion in the use of these funds; federal requirements and involvement would be minimal. The funds would be targeted for low-income populations, but states could expand coverage to higher-income populations if they wish.

Under such a program, funds for long-term-care services would be unified, divisions in funding between health and social services would be eliminated, a better balance and coordination among the full range of long-term-care services would result, and the present funding bias toward institutional care would be eliminated. States would have maximum flexibility to experiment with different approaches to meeting needs for long-term care, to set their own priorities in the use of funds to meet needs for long-term care, to integrate these services with other state programs and priorities, to adapt their approaches to local conditions and preferences, to substitute lower-cost services for higher-cost services, to better control the utilization of services, to rationalize the procurement and reimbursement of services, to relate these functions to controlling the quality of care, and to allocate services on the basis of the assessment of individual needs free from arbitrary, externally imposed constraints. There would be strong incentives to meet individual needs for care and to obtain services from providers at the lowest cost consistent with standards of quality. Efficiency, equity, and effectiveness in the administration and delivery of long-term-care services would thus be improved.

The growth in federal costs for long-term care would be controlled, but the states and the elderly are likely to oppose any limits on federal funds for long-term care unless such limits were very high. Federal funds for long-term-care services would be distributed more equitably across states under such a program, but a significant amount of financial redistribution among states would take place; poorer states would gain, but richer states would lose. A hold-harmless provision (which would prohibit a state from receiving any less federal funds than they are presently receiving) would require substantially higher federal expenditures. There would be wider variations in state per capita expenditures for long-term care if state matching was required than if it was not. A great potential for wide variations in benefits and in access to care, both across and within states, would still exist. States could either expand or restrict coverage. With no individual entitlement, certain individuals would not necessarily be assured of certain minimal services. Gaps in service coverage could also result if state long-term-care benefits and national health insurance benefits did not mesh. If the level of federal funds appropriated was too low, many needs for care would go unmet. States might choose to "underserve" rather than "overinstitutionalize." They would be free to choose, or may be forced to utilize, lower-quality services. There would be less assurance that quality standards would be maintained or improved. Separate sets of providers could develop, one set certified under less strict state standards for long-term-care services and the other set certified under stricter federal standards under national health insurance.

Pollak concludes that this option would be "an inappropriate choice—except as a complement to, for example, an interim Medicaid program" (p. 52). HEW (1976) chooses this option, but HEW (1978) states that such a major redistribution of federal funds to states for long-term care should only be considered in conjunction with national health insurance, which would offer significant fiscal relief to states for acute care.

Specialization of Program Funding for Long-Term Care by Type of Care Setting

HEW (1974), Correia (1976), and HEW (1978) discuss this kind of option. HEW (1974) and Correia propose an open-ended, individual entitlement (insurance) program for institutional long-term-care services and a separate program of closed-ended grants to states for noninstitutional long-term-care services. The first program could be administered either by the federal government or by the states. In either case, the federal government would specify nationally uniform-eligibility criteria; anyone medically certified to need institutional (SNF, ICF) care under these criteria would be entitled to receive unlimited benefits (subject to cost-sharing requirements). There would be no enrollment or premium payments; the program would be financed out of general revenues. The second program would be administered by the states. There would be no individual entitlement to services; states would determine their own eligibility criteria for benefits. Funds under this program could be used for any health or social service in noninstitutional settings but could not be used to pay for the costs of room and board. Clients would pay for room-and-board costs out of their own resources; cash-assistance payments to recipients would be maintained in full in any noninstitutional setting. Anyone meeting the eligibility criteria of both programs would be allowed to choose between institutional and noninstitutional care. State matching would be required under both programs, but the rate would be significantly higher under the program for institutional services than under the program for noninstitutional services; this would provide states with a strong fiscal incentive to develop alternatives to institutional care and to attract clients away from institutional care.

Such a system of structuring program funding for long-term care would guarantee access to institutional care for those who need it, while expanding the availability and coverage of noninstitutional care. The individual's range of choice of care settings would thus be expanded. Eligibility criteria, cost-sharing requirements, and quality standards for institutional care would be the same in all states. The use of cost-sharing schedules for institutional care would allow individuals to receive coverage without first impoverishing themselves, would encourage individuals to choose efficient providers of care, and would reduce overutilization of such services. The utilization of institutional services for care would decline, and the utilization of noninstitutional services for care would rise. In addition, direct competition would occur between the two programs, especially if the program for institutional services was federally administered and the program for noninstitutional services was state administered. Two separate systems of care would develop, providing overlapping benefits and expanding individual choice.

Expenditures for institutional care would remain open-ended, however, and both the public and the state shares of these costs would increase. If states found their share of these costs too burdensome, they might fail to assure adequate provision of institutional services and might still refuse to develop alternatives. States would be "responsible for directing persons to various care settings. In practice, they may limit any real choice for disabled persons" (HEW 1974, p. 46). Patients' representatives might become necessary to ensure patient rights to care and choice of care. Some persons may also choose "care in a setting which society will not feel is adequate" (HEW 1974, p. 45). Like all matching programs, some states may take full advantage of these programs, while other states may make relatively little use of these programs. Strong federal incentives and differentiated matching rates by state may be needed to assure more adequate and uniform provision of both types of services across states.

HEW (1978) considers two other variants of this kind of option. Under one, federal expenditures for institutional long-term care would be capped under Medicaid and the projected savings would be channeled through closed-ended grants to states for noninstitutional long-term-care services. (Federal expenditures for noninstitutional long-term-care services under Medicaid would presumably either remain open-ended or would also be channeled through the closed-ended grants to states for noninstitutional services.) This would reduce the present bias toward institutional care under Medicaid and would channel resources for community services through a more appropriate program. A cap on federal Medicaid expenditures for institutional long-term care would limit federal costs, but would "not necessarily assure the delivery of appropriate services" (HEW 1978, Appendix 6, p. 2). Since states would have to devote a higher proportion of their own resources to institutional long-term care, less of their resources would be available for community-based long-term-care services. Both the states and the elderly are likely to strongly oppose any such cap on federal expenditures for institutional long-term care, unless, perhaps, it is accompanied by a substantial increase in federal resources, because growing numbers of the elderly will increase the utilization of institutional services greatly over time. Even large expenditures on community-based care may not lower rates of institutionalization to any significant degree.

Under the second variant of this option considered by HEW (1978), federal matching rates for institutional long-term-care services under Medicaid would simply be reduced (instead of being capped), and the matching rates for noninstitutional long-term-care services under Medicaid would be raised. (This feature might also be accompanied by an expansion of Medicaid benefits for additional community and in-home services.) States would likely support any increase in federal matching rates for community-based services but would oppose any reduction in matching rates for institutional services. In addition, "there is no guarantee that the states would respond" to the differential matching rates as desired (HEW 1978, Appendix 6, p. 3). "It is highly likely that increased use and availability of community-based services would represent additional expenditures and would not be offset by reductions in the institutional population" (HEW 1978, Appendix 6, p. 3).

Specialization of Program Funding for Long-Term Care, by Type of Need or Cost

HEW (1974) and Joe and Meltzer (1976) propose a program of this nature. According to HEW (1974), a national health insurance program would cover the total costs of care in hospitals and skilled nursing facilities and (only) the costs of health services in all other care settings (including intermediate-care facilities). Individuals themselves would pay the living costs in all settings, except hospitals and skilled nursing facilities, out of their own resources or from cash-assistance payments (such as SSI). Social support services in all settings, except hospitals and skilled nursing facilities, would be covered at the option of each state through a special social services program (such as Title XX), through a state supplementation to SSI, and/or through a residual Medicaid program. Intermediate care facilities would be allowed to contract out for the provision of both health and social services. If they do so, they would simply become a special type of residence regulated under state housing codes. Ceilings would be set, however, on resident payments to intermediate care facilities for living costs and residents would be allowed to receive state supplementation and postpayment case allowances under SSI.

The Joe and Meltzer (1976) proposal differs from the HEW (1974) proposal in only a few ways. In skilled nursing facilities, Medicare, Medicaid, or a national health insurance program would only cover the costs of medical services (instead of total costs), and other programs would cover the nonmedical costs. Instead of relying on cash assistance programs to cover residential-living costs, a separate, new federal program would be created to cover the costs of room and board in all long-term-care facilities ("from SNFs to custodial domiciliary homes") (p. 24). "Flexible prospective reimbursement rates . . . would be established with regional and/or community variations to reflect cost of living and cost of housing" (p. 25).

Benefits would be scaled according to income. The costs of social and other supportive services in any setting would be covered by such programs (appropriately amended) as "Title XX, VR [Vocational Rehabilitation], Mental Health, and/or other sources of services funding at the state, local, and community level" (pp. 24-25).

Although their proposals are very similar, HEW (1974) and Joe and Meltzer (1976) each makes a different set of points about such a method of structuring program funding for long-term care. HEW (1974) states that such an approach "relies upon individual entitlement but allows state flexibility for social services" (p. 53). It assures that health care programs do in fact purchase health care and that more appropriate programs are used to meet related social and economic needs. It would broaden the spectrum of noninstitutional services and thus enhance individual choice of care settings. The budgets for all three components of long-term care would be open-ended. "Interstate variations in health care benefits would be eliminated but would continue for social support services and SSI supplementation for institutional-living allowances" (p. 54). Intermediate care facilities would be dealt with more realistically and more in accordance with their true nature. The development of "coalitions of services and/or multiservice centers" would be encouraged (p. 54). Currently autonomous care settings would be tied together into a system of care, and coordination of long-term care would be improved. Contracting out for health care services in "group residential settings is a more efficient and effective means of providing health care than" having each facility provide its own system of care (p. 54). Health care service providers would be federally certified, while social service providers would be certified by the states. In order to assure proper equilibrium among the three components of long-term care for each individual, adequate coordination and funding of each of the three components is needed; one component cannot compensate for the insufficiency of another.

Joe and Meltzer (1976) state that "separating out room and board from service costs . . . enables a much simpler, more efficient way of setting room-and-board rates that are realistically related to local conditions, zoning requirements, and costs of housing" (p. 24). "It would provide greater opportunity for alternative room and board and service arrangements, more equitable rate setting for room and board which would reflect local cost-of-living variations as well as insuring accountability for both room and board and service provision" (p. 25). Level-of-care status and reimbursement rates would be tied to individuals instead of facilities. This "would make it possible to provide for a continuum of care tailored to individual client needs" (p. 25). Facility rates would be based on individual service utilization. Intergovernmental responsibilities would be fixed more clearly. The federal government would be responsible for institutional room and board costs for those eligible for that program and for medical costs under Medicare, under national health insurance, or in conjunction with the states, under Medicaid. States and localities would be responsible for the costs of other services under Title XX, mental health, and other programs. Phasing-in would be desirable. Private care would not be excluded. "Uniform cost-accounting systems (which can provide the necessary data on costs in relation to units of service), uniform record keeping, and a computerized tracking system" would be essential (p. 26).

Local Long-Term-Care Organizations

The use of local long-term-care organizations is discussed by Correia (1976), HEW (1976), and HEW (1978). Such organizations would receive federal/state grants to provide long-term-care services in their local area. Their functions would include individual needs assessment; referral to and coordination of appropriate services; case management; planning a comprehensive, local service delivery system for long-term care (if public); quality assurance; and advocacy.

Many possible variants of such an agency exist. According to Correia (1976), such an agency could be used for noninstitutional care only or for both institutional and noninstitutional care. According to HEW (1978), they could be designed to have no power of enforcement, limited veto power, partial control of service funding, or total control of service funding. In each community, such agencies each could specialize in a certain subpopulation or each could be an HMO-type organization with particular enrollees. Providers could receive grants or be reimbursed on a fee-for-service basis or on a capitation basis. Both medical and social services could be covered or only medical services alone.

The use of local long-term-care organizations would allow much greater flexibility in allocating resources, both among individuals and among various types of services (institutional and noninstitutional, health and social), in meeting individual needs for care in responding to local needs, circumstances, preferences, and priorities, and in controlling expenditures. Fewer externally imposed constraints and control mechanisms would be needed, such as those involving restrictions on benefit coverage, eligibility criteria, reimbursement methods and rates, and various means of controlling the utilization of services. The quality of care provided would be better controlled. Individual needs assessment would provide a better basis for planning community long-term-care-service-delivery systems.

HEW (1978) points out, however, that such an approach "assumes that valid and reliable diagnostic methodologies exist or can be developed" (Appendix 1, p.7). Not everyone believes this to be so. In addition, Correia

(1976) notes that, historically, grants to such agencies have resulted in well-developed programs in some areas, but only poorly developed programs in other areas.

HEW (1978) makes few remarks about this option in general, but gives fairly extensive consideration to three specific suboptions. Under the *first* suboption, a "single regional agency would handle all public-sector LTC [long-term-care] responsibilities." (Appendix 1, p. 3). "The agency would have some authority (though not complete authority) over the use of public funds for LTC [long-term-care]. . . ." (Appendix 1, p. 4). Under the *second* suboption, the federal government would encourage the development of HMO-type organizations for long-term care of the elderly (only). Program funds would be used for capitation payments for enrollees. Under the *third* suboption, public long-term-care agencies would only serve the elderly, perhaps as extensions of area agencies on aging. They "would have direct control over service-delivery funds" and could reallocate funds from institutional care to noninstitutional care (Appendix 1, p. 7). If area agencies on aging were used, they would be linked to "skilled-service units," which would provide "socio-medical diagnostic services" (Appendix 1, p. 12).

HEW (1978) makes many points about these three suboptions.

1. They would provide a more comprehensive, coordinated, integrated, systematized, and efficient approach to long-term care, from assessment to service delivery. Consolidation of all gatekeeping to a single local point under suboption one would improve accessibility. Suboption three would represent an investment in fundamentally restructuring the service-delivery system for long-term care. Communities would be able to plan more rationally for their long-term-care needs.

2. For suboption one, HEW (1978) states that with "no direct control over most service funds, . . . gaps may exist between services needed and services provided" (Appendix 1, p. 5). However, for suboption two, it states that "no gaps should exist between services needed and services provided, as there would be complete integration between assessment and service delivery" (Appendix 1, p. 6).

3. The utilization of all long-term-care services would be controlled and inappropriate utilization and placement reduced. Stricter gatekeeping should lower the occupancy rates of intermediate care facilities. For suboption two, however, quality may be compromised in order to hold down costs. Mechanisms may be needed to monitor or assure quality and to prevent "underutilization."

4. For suboptions one and three, "through the incorporation of social workers and other nonphysicians into the diagnosis and assessment process, the medical model would be replaced" (Appendix 1, p. 7). Physicians, however, will object to relinquishing control over patient assessment, referral, and placement to nonphysicians such as social workers. For suboption

two, "some providers (especially institutional providers) might object to the HMO concept, fearing the consequences of a greater reliance on community-based services" (Appendix 1, p. 11).

5. Federal costs are estimated to be $550 million for suboption one, at least $2 billion for suboption two, and $500 million for suboption three. If a scaled-down version of suboption three is chosen using area agencies on aging, federal costs are estimated to grow from $171 million in FY 1980 to $773 million in FY 1982. The effect of suboptions one and three on private-sector costs and on provider costs is considered to be negligible. The effect of each of the three suboptions on the costs to individuals and families with needs for long-term care is also considered to be negligible. Under suboption two, individuals would achieve substantial cost savings as a result of changing from payment on a fee-for-service basis to payment on a capitation basis.

6. Politically, there may be objections to the added federal costs of the three suboptions. For suboption one, advocacy groups may prefer to have such agencies specialized by population type. Suboptions two and three should be supported by congressional committees on aging as a means of improving, and making more comprehensive, the care of the elderly. However, under these two suboptions, groups other than the elderly "may (in reality and/or in perception) receive second-class LTC" (Appendix 1, pp. 6, 7). Advocacy groups for the nonelderly "may object to concentrating on the LTC needs of the elderly" only and may contend "that once the LTC needs of the elderly are met, the needs of the other groups may be ignored or forgotten" (Appendix 1, p. 11). Suboption three "would help to fulfill departmental commitments to undertake a major aging initiative as part of the reauthorization of the OAA [Older Americans Act]" (p. 15). It would appeal to aging constituencies but not to other constituencies. However, elderly advocacy groups may prefer to have the fiscal resources used instead for expanding Medicare benefits.

7. Suboptions one and three would put limited fiscal resources into expensive, new administrative structures rather than into expanding services. it would be difficult for these new agencies to coordinate if no services were available. Suboption two would require "substantial new federal administrative structures . . . for implementation" (Appendix 1, p. 6).

8. Suboption one would make it possible to target the use of any expansion in long-term-care benefits to the most cost effective cases. Suboption two would result in a significant expansion of existing services, "whereas suboption three calls for a limited expansion of existing services" (Appendix 1, p. 8). Suboptions two and three would cover many more elderly persons and services than do present programs.

9. If many social services were covered under suboption two, the necessary capitation rates would be "prohibitively expensive." (Appendix 1,

p. 5). "The supply of LTC [long-term care] would be inceased [only] to the extent [that] organization capacity developed in response to capitation payments" (Appendix 1, p. 6). A sufficient supply of such HMO-type organizations may not develop "in response to the availability of the capitation payments" (Appendix 1, p. 6). "A 'liberal' capitation rate may be necessary in order to encourage the development of HMO-type long-term-care organizations" (Appendix 1, p. 9).

10. Agencies developed under suboption two or three for the elderly could serve as prototypes for later expansion to populations with long-term-care needs other than the elderly. However, if area agencies on aging were expanded to provide services to the nonelderly (under suboption three), the nonelderly may resent assessment and placement by agencies whose main focus is on the needs of the elderly.

11. Under suboption one, jurisdictional conflicts could arise between such agencies and regional health planning agencies. Under suboptions one and three, the ambiguity of the relationship between such an agency and existing agencies and service providers may make such proposals administratively difficult to implement. Existing programs and providers may object to giving such new agencies any authority over long-term-care services.

12. Suboption three "can build directly upon existing agencies (e.g., the area aging agencies)" (Appendix 1, p. 7) and "can be achieved within the context of the authority of the Older Americans Act" (Appendix 1, p. 14). Linkages can be developed with existing health complexes to provide primary health care services. "It is unclear [however] whether the area agencies on aging are the best vehicle through which to develop" local long-term-care organizations (Appendix 1, p. 14). They "are sometimes weak organizationally and may not be capable of handling these new functions. In addition, AAAs have not tended to develop strong working relationships with health delivery agencies and could have difficulty assuring that needed health services are provided" (Appendix 1, p. 15).

This review has covered only those options that were included in earlier analyses. For those options that have been presented in this volume, the details as well as the impact of the options have been greatly expanded. Still other options exist which have not been incorporated in this volume or in previous analyses.

Notes

1. W. Pollak, "Federal Long-Term Care Strategy: Options and Analysis" (Washington, D.C.: Urban Institute, 17 October 1973, revised 25 February 1974). Reprinted with permission.

2. T. Joe and J. Meltzer, "Policies and Strategies for Long-Term Care" (San Francisco: Health Policy Program, University of California, 14 May 1976). Reprinted with permission.

References

Congressional Budget Office (CBO), 1977. *Long-Term Care for the Elderly and Disabled*. Washington, D.C., February; *Long-Term Care: Actuarial Cost Estimates*. August.

Correia, E. 1976. "National Health Insurance, Welfare Reform, and the Disabled: Issues in Program Reform," Prepared for Office of the Assistant Secretary for Planning and Evaluation, U.S. Department of Health, Education, and Welfare, Washington, D.C., August.

Joe, T. and Meltzer, J. 1976. "Policies and Strategies for Long-Term Care." San Francisco: Health Policy Program, University of California, May 14.

Pollak, W. 1974. "Federal Long-Term Care Strategy: Options and Analysis." Washington, D.C.: The Urban Institute, 17 October 1973, revised 25 February 1974.

U.S. Department of Health, Education, and Welfare, 1974. "Program Design Choices for Long-Term Care Legislative Initiative—Decision Memorandum," Office of the Secretary, Washington, D.C., August.

_____ . 1976. "Long-Term Care Services Legislative Proposal." Office of the Secretary, Washington, D.C., October 19.

_____ . 1978. "Memorandum for July 14, 1978, Briefing, Major Initiative: Long-Term-Care/Community Services," Office of the Secretary, Washington, D.C.

Index

Home-care services: *(cont.)* allowance,
95, 103, 108, 111; and eligibility, 46; expenditures for, 14-15; and federal
government, 16; and insurance, 65, 68,
75, 76, 89-90; and Medicare, 15, 61,
103, 104, 113; versus nursing homes, 26,
97; quality, 16; and PCOs, 195; and
S/HMOs, 202, 209, 211; and Title XX,
16, 61
Home health agencies, 4, 11, 153, 164,
199
Home health aides, 4, 26, 210
Homemaker services, 15, 26, 186, 231;
and disability allowance, 95, 97, 100,
109, 113, 115; and insurance, 75; and
S/HMOs, 202, 204, 210; and single
agency, 164, 176
Hospitals, 185, 186; and case management,
153; cost of care, 108; and HMOs, 191,
193; long-term population, 11; and
PCOs, 196, 197; and S/HMOs, 204; and
systems model, 231, 232
Housing: demand, 47; and disability
allowance, 106, 109-110; funds, 46, 61;
and insurance, 65, 67, 68, 70, 75, 83;
and long-term care, 106, 109-110
Hurtado, A., 193

Implementation, 39-41, 43-44, 144, 146
Implementation (Pressman and Wildavsky),
144
Income: and bloc grant, 51, 55; ceilings,
83, 87, 91; and disability, 63-64; and
eligibility, 18, 30, 55, 61, 71, 101-102,
108, 109, 177, 181, 189; and insurance,
69, 73, 77, 82, 83, 86-88; and single
agency, 175
Income assistance programs, 185. *See also*
Supplemental Security Income
Incrementalism, 11, 160-161, 176
Indiana, 177
Individualization of service, 131, 140,
151, 155
Inflation, 7, 64, 68-70, 73, 205
Institutionalization: bias toward, 4, 7, 12,
14-15, 54, 71, 79-80, 87, 159, 185-186,
242; costs, 14, 15, 17-18, 46, 87, 88,
113, 119, 150, 152, 185, 243-244; and
disability allowance, 97; and insurance,
23, 24, 75, 76; and quality of care, 16-17
Insurance: and acute care, 74; administrative costs, 70, 73, 90-91; benefits, 5,
63-67, 70, 86, 88; and family, 64, 69-70,
73, 74; group, 72; and inflation, 64,
69-70, 73; and institutionalization, 23,
24, 75, 76; payments, 5, 63, 66-67, 69,
72, 83; premiums, 66, 69, 71-72, 73;

and S/HMOs, 201. *See also* National
health insurance
Interest groups, 11, 39-40
Intergovernmental Cooperation Act of
1968, 32
Intermediate care facilities (ICFs), 14,
46, 240, 245, 248

Joe, T., 23, 237, 239, 241, 245-246

Kaiser Plan, 191, 193, 194

La Vor, J., 167
Legal services, 164, 177, 227
Lennox, K., 191
Lescohier, I.H., 165
Local agencies, 19-20, 24-25, 171, 181,
209, 247-250. *See also* Single agency
Longevity, 11
Los Angeles, 191
Lynn, L.E., Jr., 147

Madison, James, 42
Massachusetts, 124, 164, 180, 181
Mayhew, D., 44
Meals services, 67, 78, 113, 176, 178
Means tests, 97, 101-102, 108, 175, 177,
180-181; *See also* Income
Medicaid: and acute care, 47; and copayment, 109; costs, 56, 196; and day-care
centers, 179; eligibility, 18, 45, 61, 71,
87, 96, 101, 181; expenditures for long-
term care, 16, 18-19, 46, 49, 51, 195,
244-245, 247; and fragmentation, 20;
and HMOs, 199; and home health care,
14-15, 71, 103; and income, 71; and
institutionalization, 14-15, 16, 18, 71;
and national health insurance, 85, 88;
and nursing homes, 16, 18-19, 50, 61-62,
102, 191; and PCOs, 194, 195; and providers, 52; reimbursement rates, 17, 46,
171; restrictions, 15; and S/HMOs, 200,
201, 202; and single agency, 171; and
states, 14-15, 17, 23, 29, 47, 61, 106,
186, 203, 211, 225; and systems management model, 225
Medical Aid to the Aged, 3
Medicare, 3; and disability allowance, 103,
110; eligibility, 45, 61-62, 96; expenditures for long-term care, 46, 186, 247;
and HMOs, 190-194, 198, 199, 204-205,
206; and home health services, 15, 61,
103, 104, 113; and nursing homes, 16,
61-62, 245; and PCOs, 194; restrictions,
46; and S/HMOs, 198, 200, 201, 202,
204, 206; and single agency, 171; and
states, 106

About the Authors

Dennis F. Beatrice, M.P.A., was a research associate at the Center for Health Policy Analysis and Research at Brandeis University from 1978 to 1979. He is currently director of the Long-Term Care Unit, Medicaid Division, Department of Public Welfare, in Massachusetts.

David E. Berman, M.S.W., is a research associate at the Center for Health Policy Analysis and Research. He is currently a doctoral candidate at the Florence Heller Graduate School for Advanced Studies in Social Welfare, Brandeis University.

Christine E. Bishop, Ph.D., is an assistant professor in the Economics Department at Boston University School of Management and a senior research associate at the Center for Health Policy Analysis and Research.

Larry M. Diamond, M.A., is a project associate at the University Health Policy Consortium at Brandeis University and instructor at Boston University School of Medicine and Boston University School of Social Work.

Leonard W. Gruenberg, Ph.D., is a senior research associate at the University Health Policy Consortium's Long-Term Care Unit at Brandeis University. Dr. Gruenberg was formerly affiliated with the Department of Social Gerontological Research at the Hebrew Rehabilitation Center for the Aged.

Robert B. Hudson, Ph.D., is assistant professor of politics and social welfare at the Florence Heller Graduate School for Advanced Studies in Social Welfare, Brandeis University. Dr. Hudson is also affiliated with the Center for Health Policy Analysis and Research.

Robert Morris, D.S.W., is Kirstein Professor of Social Planning at the Florence Heller Graduate School for Advanced Studies in Social Welfare, Brandeis University, and lecturer at Harvard University School of Public Health. For six years he served as the director of the Levinson Policy Institute at Brandeis University.

Karl A. Pillemer, M.A., is a research assistant at the Center for Health Policy Analysis and Research and a doctoral candidate in sociology at Brandeis University.

Paul Youket, M.A., M.C.P., is a research assistant at the Center for Health Policy Analysis and Research. Mr. Youket is seeking candidacy for a doctorate at the Florence Heller Graduate School for Advanced Studies in Social Welfare at Brandeis University.

About the Editors

James J. Callahan, Jr., is director of the Levinson Policy Institute and deputy director of the University Health Policy Center. He was formerly the Secretary of the Department of Elder Affairs for the Commonwealth of Massachusetts and was responsible for overseeing the services to the elderly in Massachusetts, including those funded by the Older Americans Act and by Title XX of the Social Security Act. Dr. Callahan previously served as the superintendent of the Massachusetts Hospital School, a 150-bed facility for physically handicapped young people, and was also superintendent of the Lemuel Shattuck Chronic Disease Hospital in Boston for six months during his tenure at the Hospital School. Dr. Callahan has also served as a member of the Massachusetts Rate-Setting Commission and was director of the state's Medicaid program from 1969 to 1971. He received the A.B. from the College of the Holy Cross, the M.S.W. from Boston College, and the Ph.D. from the Florence Heller Graduate School for Advanced Studies in Social Welfare, Brandeis University. Dr. Callahan is the author of numerous articles and is the producer-host for a television program directed toward older persons titled "Senior Circuit."

Stanley S. Wallack is currently the director of the Center for Health Policy Analysis and Research and the University Health Policy Consortium. An economist, he has taught at the University of Illinois in Champaign/Urbana. From 1970 to 1977, he worked on major health policy issues for the federal government in both the executive and legislative branches. Dr. Wallack's last federal appointment was as deputy assistant director for health, income assistance, and veterans affairs at the Congressional Budget Office, where he was responsible for producing legislative and budget-options papers for Senate and House committees. He has published papers on a wide array of health policy issues from hospital-cost containment to mental health.